D1192562

Diabetic Dream Desserts

Sandra Woodruff, RD

Avery Publishing Group

Garden City Park, New York

Text Illustrator: John Wincek
Front Cover Photograph: John Strange
Cover Design: William Gonzalez
Typesetting: Bonnie Freid
In-House Editor: Joanne Abrams

Cataloging-in-Publication Data
Woodruff, Sandra L.
    Diabetic dream desserts: over 120 simple and delicious low fat/
Sandra Woodruff.
      p. cm.
    Includes index.
    ISBN 0-89529-712-4
    1. Diabetes—Diet therapy—Recipes. 2. Desserts. I. Title.
RC662.W66 1996
641.8'6—dc20   96-22093
                                              CIP

Printed in the United States of America

10 9 8 7 6

Contents

This book is dedicated to my favorite taste testers, Wiley and C.D.

Acknowledgments

It has been a great pleasure to produce this book with the talented and dedicated professionals at Avery Publishing Group, who have so generously lent their support and creativity at every stage of production. Special thanks go to Rudy Shur and Ken Rajman for providing the opportunity to publish this book, and to my editor, Joanne Abrams, whose hard work, endless patience, and diligent attention to detail have added so much.

Thanks also go to my dear friends and family members for their enduring support and encouragement, and to my clients and coworkers, whose questions and ideas keep me learning and experimenting with new things. Last, but not least, I would like to thank my husband, Tom Maureau, for his long-term support and encouragement, and for always being there for me.

Preface

In the last few years, we've all learned how a proper diet—high in whole grains and other whole foods, and low in fat and refined sugar—is necessary for good health. While important for everyone, such a diet is truly *vital* for the 14 million people who have diabetes. In fact, for 90 percent of the people with diabetes, poor nutrition was a contributing factor in the development of the disease. If this sounds impossible, consider the following: The average American derives close to half of his or her calories from fats and refined sugar. The rest of the diet often consists of refined grains and nutrient-poor processed foods. Most people eat only half the recommended amount of fruits and vegetables, and get only half the fiber needed for good health. Combine a diet like this with a sedentary lifestyle, and you have a situation ripe for the development of not just diabetes, but also obesity, heart disease, cancer, and other disorders.

The good news is that just as poor nutrition often contributes to diabetes, proper nutrition is the cornerstone of treatment for this disease. In fact, with nutritional therapy and exercise, people can help control and sometimes even reverse their diabetes. *Diabetic Dream Desserts* can help you get started. This book allows you to maximize your nutrition and still enjoy great-tasting sweet treats. From Cinnamon Carrot Cake, to Sensational Strawberry Pie, to Polenta Pudding, to Chocolate Pecan Biscotti, every recipe has been designed to eliminate or greatly reduce fat and sugar, to increase fiber, and to boost nutrition. Just as important, every recipe has been kitchen-tested to make sure that you enjoy success each and every time you make it, and people-tested to make sure that every treat you create is a hit.

Diabetic Dream Desserts begins by explaining just how sugar, fat, fiber, and other nutrients affect diabetes, and how a wise diet can contribute to good health. You'll then learn how to use whole grain flours, fruits, fruit juices, spices, natural sweeteners, and natural fat substitutes to create wholesome and delicious treats that will help you maximize nutrition. You'll also learn how to make the best use of artificial sweeteners in recipes. The remainder of the book presents a fabulous selection of delectable cakes, pies, puddings, cookies, cobblers, crisps, dessert breads, and other sweet treats—each made with wholesome ingredients, with little or no added fat, and with a lot less refined sugar than that used in most traditional desserts.

In addition to including tried-and-true recipes, *Diabetic Dream Desserts* provides a wealth of tips to guide you in creating more healthful versions of your own favorite treats. Within these pages you will discover how to reduce or eliminate sugar, how to use natural fat substitutes, how to use many of the new reduced-fat and nonfat products, and how to use whole grain flours in your favorite desserts. These simple tips will make modifying your own recipes a breeze.

So take out your spatula, and get ready to learn just how healthy *and* delicious desserts can be. It is my hope that *Diabetic Dream Desserts* will prove to you that treats do not have to be full of fat and sugar, and that wholesome goodies can be satisfying, exciting, and fun.

Introduction

Making and eating great food is one of life's simplest and greatest pleasures. And homemade desserts usually top the list of favorites. Cookies fresh from the oven, bubbling cobblers and fruit crisps, warm and yeasty coffee cakes and buns, and sweet and delicious cakes and pies have warmed the hearts of generations. Homemade treats are also a special part of many family traditions as treasured recipes are passed from parent to child with loving care. Just the aroma of freshly baked cookies, breads, cakes, and other treats can bring back memories of special times.

For many years, people with diabetes were mistakenly told that sweets were strictly off limits; thus, diabetic dessert books totally avoided the use of sugar. Unfortunately, in the process, these books often compromised nutrition by including too much fat and too many artificial sweeteners, and by relying mainly on refined flours.

More recent research has shown that people with diabetes *can* incorporate moderate amounts of sugar into their diets and still maintain good blood sugar control. Thus, *Diabetic Dream Desserts* is very different from earlier cookbooks.

This unique collection of recipes was designed to help you create delicious treats that are low in sugar, fat, and refined foods, and surprisingly high in the nutrients needed for good health.

As a nutritionist and teacher, and as a person who loves good food, I long ago began looking for ways to improve the healthfulness of dishes. My first step was to reduce or totally eliminate the fat in foods. At the same time, though, I discovered that many of the natural fat substitutes I used reduced the need for sugar. As the result of years of experimentation and kitchen testing, and of many helpful suggestions from clients and students, I developed simple ways to make moist and flavorful cakes, cookies, pies, cobblers, puddings, and other treats with little or no fat and a lot less sugar. These discoveries are what I am sharing in this book. Besides eliminating or reducing fat and sugar, I have further improved the nutritional value of desserts and sweet treats by using whole grains and whole grain flours. The result? Great-tasting desserts that can be easily incorporated into any diabetic diet.

One of the nicest features of this book is the

simplicity of the recipes. Every effort has been made to keep the number of ingredients to a minimum and to utilize as few pots, pans, equipment, and utensils as possible. Many of the recipes can be easily mixed by hand in only one bowl.

And many of these recipes are also easy enough for beginners. So get your whole family involved—these desserts are *not* just for diabetics—and let *Diabetic Dream Desserts* be the start of some wonderful memories.

1

Having Your Cake and Eating It, Too

Sometimes, you can have your cake and eat it too . . . and your pies, cobblers, crisps, puddings, and cookies. This book presents recipes for a variety of delectable desserts prepared in accordance with the latest diabetic guidelines. All of these recipes contain low to moderate amounts of sugar and are greatly reduced in fat. Many also incorporate wholesome whole grains, fruits, and other fiber-rich foods. Experienced cooks and novices alike will be amazed by the number of creative and healthful ways in which fat and sugar can be reduced in sweet treats.

This chapter begins by explaining what diabetes is, and how sugar, fat, fiber, and other nutrients affect this largely preventable and treatable disorder. You'll learn why a low-fat, high-fiber eating plan is usually the wisest choice, and how certain vitamins and minerals can help your body handle sugar more efficiently. Following this, you will learn about the various ingredients used in recipes throughout this book—ingredients that will allow you to prepare healthful treats that are low in fat and sugar, and high in satisfaction.

DIABETES AND YOUR DIET

In simple terms, diabetes is a disorder that causes blood sugar concentrations to become abnormally high. This disease centers on the hormone insulin, and on the way in which the body metabolizes food.

Eating sets off a complex series of events. As the food moves from the mouth to the stomach to the intestines, it is systematically broken down, and its carbohydrates, proteins, and fats are released. As sugar enters the bloodstream in the form of glucose, blood sugar levels rise. At this point, the pancreas normally secretes insulin, which transports sugar from the blood into the cells. There, it can be used for energy. But when someone has diabetes, either the pancreas does not make enough insulin to handle dietary sugar, or the cells do not respond to the insulin. As a result, the sugar stays in the blood instead of entering the cells, and the cells become starved for energy. People who do not control their diabetes have chronically elevated blood sugar levels.

Over a number of years, this can lead to serious complications.

Ninety percent of the people who get diabetes develop the disease during adulthood—usually past the age of forty. Of these people, the vast majority are overweight, consume diets high in fat and refined foods, and lead sedentary lives. The good news is that positive changes in nutrition and exercise are often all that is needed to keep diabetes in check. The following sections describe how various nutrients affect diabetes, and how you can make these nutrients work for you.

Sugar—Just Another Carbohydrate?

The most obvious dietary change that people think of when planning a diabetic diet is the elimination of sugar. Indeed, sugar has long been discouraged in the diabetic diet, and complex carbohydrates—whole grains, for instance—have been recommended instead. This guideline has recently been revised, as research has demonstrated that most people with diabetes can include *some* sugar in their diets.

How much sugar is acceptable? For the general population, it is recommended that no more than 10 percent of caloric intake come from refined, simple sugars like white table sugar. This means that a person who needs 2,000 calories a day should limit his or her sugar intake to 50 grams—about 12½ teaspoons—a day, although less would be better. About half this amount—6 teaspoons a day—would be prudent for people with diabetes. But be sure to check with your health-care provider to learn exactly how much sugar is acceptable in your diet.

When including sugar or sugar-containing desserts in a diabetic diet, it's vital to substitute the sugar for other carbohydrates, rather than simply adding it to your meal plan. Why? The amounts and types of foods prescribed by your nutritionist or physician are related to your weight-maintenance or weight-loss goals, and to any medications you're taking, such as insulin injections or diabetes pills. Food eaten in excess of those prescribed by your meal plan can raise your blood sugar and cause weight gain.

Also keep in mind that despite the fact that the sugar allowance for diabetes has been liberalized, it is prudent to keep your sugar intake to a minimum. After all, sugar is still a nutrient-poor food. And eaten in excess, sugar can actually deplete your body of the B vitamins, chromium, and other important nutrients needed by the body to metabolize carbohydrates. Too much sugar can also raise levels of blood cholesterol and triglycerides, which are already a problem for many people with diabetes. And, of course, most sweets contain more than just sugar—fat and refined flour are usually other prominent ingredients. These foods should not be a regular part of anyone's diet.

For your convenience, every recipe in this book includes a listing of diabetic exchanges so that you can work the food into your own meal plans. Information on calories, carbohydrate, and other nutrients is also provided for people who use other diabetic meal-planning techniques, such as carbohydrate counting.

Just as important, the recipes in this book include wholesome ingredients like whole grain flours, oats, fruits, wheat germ, and low-fat and nonfat dairy products. And they contain 25 to 75 percent less sugar than traditional recipes. Ingredients like fruit juices, fruit purées, and dried fruits; flavorings and spices like vanilla, nutmeg, cinnamon, and orange rind; and mildly sweet grains like oat flour, oat bran, quick-cooking oats, and whole wheat pastry flour have been used to reduce the need for sugar.

The Role of Fat

Excess fat is the biggest problem in most people's diets—and this is true for people with diabetes, too.

High-fat diets are typically low in nutrients and fiber. They are also a primary cause of obesity. And since obesity is a strong risk factor for the development of Type II diabetes, the control of fat is especially important for people with this disease.

How does a high-fat diet promote obesity? With more than twice the calories of carbohydrate or protein, fat is a concentrated source of calories. Compare a cup of flour (almost pure carbohydrates) with a cup of butter or margarine (almost pure fat). The flour has 400 calories, while the butter has *1,600* calories. It's easy to see where most of our calories come from.

Besides being high in calories, fat is also readily converted into body fat when eaten in excess. Carbohydrate-rich foods eaten in excess are also stored as fat, but they must first be converted into fat—a process that burns up some of the carbohydrates. The bottom line is that a high-fat diet will cause 20 percent more weight gain than will a high-carbohydrate diet, even when the two diets contain the same number of calories. So a high-fat diet is a double-edged sword for the weight-conscious person. It is high in calories, and it is high in the kind of nutrient that is most readily stored as body fat.

For the person with diabetes, a high-fat diet poses a threat to much more than weight. You see, diabetes affects the way the body metabolizes fat, causing fat and cholesterol to build up in the blood more than they would accumulate in a nondiabetic person. This explains why diabetes is considered a risk factor for heart disease.

How much fat should a person with diabetes eat? For the general population, it is recommended that fat calories constitute no more than 30 percent of the diet—although 20 to 25 percent would be even better in most cases. These same guidelines apply to most people with diabetes.

Of course, people with diabetes already keep track of their fats by using one of two methods. Those who use the "Exchange Lists for Meal Planning" are allowed a certain number of fat exchanges each day. One fat exchange—the equivalent of 5 grams of fat—includes one teaspoon of butter, margarine, or mayonnaise; one tablespoon of reduced-fat butter, margarine, or mayonnaise; or one tablespoon of nuts or seeds. Fat exchanges may also be spent on fat-containing foods, such as meat, dairy products, and baked goods. When people use the other method—carbohydrate counting—to monitor their diet, they count fat grams, along with calories and carbohydrates. The number of fat grams or fat exchanges you are allowed should be determined by your nutritionist or physician based on your weight-management goals, your blood sugar level, and your levels of blood cholesterol and triglycerides.

The Role of Fiber

Dietary fiber, formerly known as roughage, is a type of complex carbohydrate found in unrefined plant foods like whole grains, whole grain flours, fruits, vegetables, and legumes (dried beans). Because fiber is resistant to digestion, it passes through the body largely unchanged. Does this mean that fiber has little effect on the body? Not at all. As fiber makes its way through the body, it has a tremendous impact. And, as you will see, fiber can be a real boon to the person with diabetes.

There are two kinds of dietary fiber: insoluble fiber and soluble fiber. Each kind offers unique health benefits.

Insoluble fiber—which is comprised of the tough, fibrous structures of the plant—does not dissolve in water. Therefore, in the intestines, insoluble fiber acts like a sponge by absorbing water and keeping the intestinal contents soft. In this way, insoluble fiber prevents constipation and diverticulosis. It also pushes wastes and carcinogens quickly through the colon, keeping it clean and disease-free.

Soluble fiber, on the other hand, readily dissolves in water. Although this fiber has little effect on the colon, it is of special importance to the person with diabetes because it can help stabilize blood sugar levels. Soluble fiber slows digestion and delays the rise in blood sugar after a meal. It also helps protect against heart disease, for which people with diabetes are at high risk. Soluble fiber reduces blood cholesterol levels by binding with bile acids, the raw materials from which cholesterol is made. As bile acids are swept from the body along with the fiber, less material is available to the body for the manufacture of cholesterol, causing blood cholesterol concentrations to drop.

Watching your weight? Fiber, like fat, provides a feeling of fullness. For this reason, fiber is especially important in a low-fat eating plan. As any dieter can tell you, a low-fat diet that includes mostly refined low-fiber foods will leave you feeling hungry. A low-fat, high-fiber eating plan, though, will keep you feeling full and satisfied. The fact that fibrous foods require more chewing and take longer to eat also makes them more satisfying.

How much fiber is sufficient for good health? For the general population, 25 to 35 grams per day is the recommended amount. Some eating plans for people with diabetes, though, may include as much as 50 grams per day. Individuals who are not used to eating high-fiber foods should add these foods to their diets gradually and drink plenty of water. Some may experience bloating and gas when they begin a high-fiber regimen, but this usually passes in a few weeks as the body becomes accustomed to eating whole, natural foods.

Fortunately, when made properly, fruit desserts, pies, cakes, cookies, and breads can be good sources of fiber. How can the fiber content of these treats be boosted? One way to increase fiber is to replace some or all of the refined flour in the recipe with a whole grain product. To show what a big difference this little change can make, see the following table, which allows you to compare the fiber content of various whole grain flours with that of refined white flour.

Fiber Content of Selected Flours

Flour 4 ounces (about 1 cup)	Fiber
Barley flour	13.6 grams
Brown rice flour	6.0 grams
Buckwheat flour	14.0 grams
Cornmeal (whole grain)	9.6 grams
Oat flour	16.0 grams
Refined (white) flour	2.8 grams
Rye flour	15.2 grams
Whole wheat flour	13.6 grams

The recipes in this book have been designed to maximize fiber—without sacrificing great taste. Many of the recipes include ingredients like whole wheat flour and wheat germ, which are rich in insoluble fiber. In other recipes, oats, oat bran, and oat flour provide soluble fiber. And fruit purées and dried fruits provide both soluble and insoluble fiber, as well as reducing the need for fat.

The Benefits of High-Fiber, Low-Fat Eating Plans

The value of a low-fat, fiber-rich diet in the treatment of diabetes became evident in the early 1970s, when Dr. James Anderson of the University of Kentucky developed the high-carbohydrate, high-fiber (HCF) diet. This low-fat eating plan—which derives only 10 to 15 percent of its calories from fats—emphasizes complex carbohydrate- and fiber-rich foods, such as whole grains, legumes, vegetables, and fruits. Lean meats and low-fat dairy products are also included, while table and cooking fats are avoided. A commonly used variation of this diet is the high-fiber maintenance (HFM) meal plan.

This is similar to the HCF diet, but allows slightly more fat—about 20 to 25 percent of total calories.

High-fiber, low-fat eating plans have worked wonders for many people with diabetes. They have been found to promote weight loss and to lower blood sugar, cholesterol, and triglyceride levels. They can even reduce or eliminate the need for insulin injections and diabetes pills.

How do HCF diets work? A variety of factors are involved in the food plan's success. For instance, fibrous whole foods like whole grains, legumes, vegetables, and fruits, are rich in nutrients such as chromium, magnesium, and zinc—nutrients that are processed out of refined foods. These nutrients help the body metabolize carbohydrates. And, as already mentioned, soluble fiber helps stabilize blood sugar levels, while both the high amount of fiber and the low amount of fat help promote weight loss.

Are low-fat diets right for everyone with diabetes? No. When someone with diabetes also has high blood cholesterol and triglycerides, a low-fat, high-carbohydrate eating plan may not bring about sufficient improvement. In addition, people with certain bowel diseases may not be able to tolerate a high-fiber, low-fat regimen. For those people who cannot follow the HCF diet, a moderate- to high-fat diet—one that derives 30 to 40 percent of its calories from fat—may be prescribed. Such a regimen avoids artery-clogging saturated fats, and instead relies on monounsaturated fats like olive oil, canola oil, nuts, and avocados. Keep in mind, though, that while monounsaturated fats are heart-healthy, they contain just as many calories as other fats. So people who tend to gain weight easily must be especially careful when following this type of plan.

Because everyone's needs are different, your physician or nutritionist will structure your eating plan according to your calorie needs and treatment goals. If you are following a low-fat, high-fiber plan, the recipes in this book, which contain little or no fat, will help you reach your goals. If your meal plan allows for more fat than the recipes in this book provide, it will be a simple matter to add a little fat at each meal. Just be sure to avoid saturated fats, and to instead choose nuts, avocados, and other foods that are rich in monounsaturated fats.

Vitamins and Minerals

Over forty nutrients are known to be essential for good health, and more are discovered all the time. Several of these nutrients merit special mention because they are important in the body's handling of blood sugar. Because many people eat highly-refined processed diets, they do not get enough of these important nutrients. A healthful, well-balanced diet is the first line of defense against nutritional deficiencies. Your physician or nutritionist may also recommend nutritional supplements as part of your treatment plan.

Chromium. This mineral works with insulin to transport glucose from the blood into the cells. When someone is chromium-deficient, insulin does not work as effectively, and blood sugar levels rise.

The recommended daily intake of chromium is 50 to 200 micrograms. Yet 90 percent of Americans are believed to consume less than even the lower recommended intake. Why is chromium so lacking in people's diets? Unprocessed carbohydrate-rich foods, like whole grains and molasses, naturally supply the chromium needed for the metabolism of these foods. When these foods are processed into refined grains and sugars, though, the chromium is removed.

How do you know if you are chromium deficient? Unfortunately, there is no easy laboratory test that can determine this. But if you take a look at your eating habits, you will get a good idea of your chromium intake. Do you eat refined grains like white rice, white bread, and other products made from refined flour, instead of whole grain products? Do you eat sugary foods on a regular basis? If the answer to these questions is "yes," you may be chromium-deficient. When you eat refined grains and sugars, you must borrow from your body's stores of chromium in order to break these foods down. When the body's stores become depleted, insulin can no longer work efficiently, and blood sugar levels rise.

The recipes in this book use ingredients like whole-grain flours, oats, bran, and wheat germ as much as possible. By using these whole foods and limiting sugar, these goodies will help keep your chromium stores intact. To further insure a good supply of chromium, be sure to also make other chromium-rich foods—molasses, brewer's yeast, prunes, nuts, seafood, and mushrooms, for instance—a regular part of your diet.

Magnesium. This mineral plays a role in the release of insulin from the pancreas, and is necessary for the breakdown of glucose in the body. Therefore, a deficiency of magnesium can contribute to high blood sugar levels. Magnesium also helps protect against heart disease and high blood pressure, which often go hand-in-hand with diabetes.

Unfortunately, people with diabetes are at a higher-than-normal risk for magnesium deficiency, since diabetics with poorly controlled blood sugar lose a higher-than-normal amount of magnesium in their urine. In fact, researchers estimate that 25 percent of people with diabetes may be magnesium deficient. Certain diuretics—taken by many people with diabetes—can also cause magnesium to be lost from the body.

To make matters worse, many people do not consume enough magnesium. You see, like chromium, magnesium is processed out of foods. A healthful, balanced diet of whole foods, though, can help insure that you get enough of this impor-

tant mineral. Good magnesium sources include whole grains, bran cereals, nuts and seeds, bananas, legumes, and green vegetables.

Zinc. Because insulin is stored in zinc crystals in the pancreas, zinc has an important role in the control of blood sugar levels. This mineral is also involved in many aspects of carbohydrate metabolism. Good zinc status is also essential for a healthy immune system and for proper wound healing—important considerations for people with diabetes, who tend to have slow-healing cuts.

Like magnesium, zinc may be excreted in the urine as the result of certain diuretics. And, like both magnesium and chromium, zinc is lost during the refining of grains. So a healthful, whole foods diet can help supply the zinc you need for good health, just as it can provide other valuable nutrients. The richest sources of this mineral include seafood (especially oysters), lean meats, whole grains, and legumes.

Antioxidants. Antioxidants include vitamin E, vitamin C, and carotenoids such as beta-carotene, lycopene, lutein, alpha-carotene, and many others. In addition, the minerals selenium, copper, and zinc are essential for the production of some enzymes that function as antioxidants.

Antioxidants are of special importance to people with diabetes, as they squelch the destructive free radicals, which can promote diabetic complications such as heart and vascular disease. But like the nutrients previously discussed, antioxidants are in short supply in many diets. Why? Vitamin E, like many other nutrients, is processed out of foods. In addition, people who consume large amounts of polyunsaturated fats—like those in refined vegetable oils, margarine, and mayonnaise—have increased requirements for this nutrient. A diet that is rich in whole grains and includes moderate amounts of nuts, seeds, and wheat germ helps provide the antioxidant nutrient vitamin E, as well as minerals like selenium, copper, and zinc, which are essential for the production of antioxidant enzymes.

As for vitamin C and the carotenoids, fresh fruits and vegetables are the best source of these nutrients. Unfortunately, most people eat only half of the recommended five or more servings a day.

As you have just seen, sugar is not the only factor that is important when planning a diabetic diet. Fat, fiber, and many other nutrients also must be considered in the management of diabetes. In the remainder of this section, you will become acquainted with the healthful ingredients that will help you prune the sugar and fat from your diet, and maximize the fiber, vitamins, and minerals.

ABOUT THE INGREDIENTS

The recipes in this book will allow you to make goodies that not only are delicious, but will work well in your meal plan. In the pages that follow, we'll take a look at the wholesome grains, flours, sweeteners, and other ingredients that can help make virtually any dessert a dream.

Low-Fat and Nonfat Dairy Products

A wide range of nonfat and low-fat dairy products are available, making it possible to create deceptively rich cheesecakes, parfaits, puddings, and dessert fillings. Here are some of the dairy products used throughout this book.

Buttermilk. Buttermilk adds a rich flavor and texture to baked goods like biscuits, muffins, and cakes, and lends a "cheesy" taste to cheesecakes. Originally a by-product of butter making, this product should perhaps be called "butterless" milk. Most brands of buttermilk contain from 0.5 to 2 percent fat by weight, but some brands contain as much as 3.5 percent fat. Choose brands that contain no more than 1 percent milkfat.

If you do not have buttermilk on hand, a good substitute can be made by mixing equal parts of nonfat yogurt and skim milk. Alternatively, place a tablespoon of vinegar or lemon juice in a one-cup measure, and fill to the one-cup mark with skim milk. Let the mixture sit for five minutes before using.

Cream Cheese. Regular full-fat cream cheese contains 10 grams of fat per ounce, making this popular spread a real menace if you're trying to reduce dietary fat. A tasty alternative is light cream cheese, which has only 5 grams of fat per ounce. Another reduced-fat alternative is Neufchâtel cheese, which contains 6 grams of fat per ounce. And, of course, nonfat cream cheese contains no fat at all. Like light cream cheese and Neufchâtel, nonfat cream cheese may be used in cheesecakes, frostings, and dessert fillings. Look for brands like Philadelphia Free and Healthy Choice.

When making cheesecakes, keep in mind that nonfat cream cheese—especially the soft tub type—has a higher moisture content than reduced-fat and full-fat brands. For this reason, cheesecakes made with nonfat brands may have a watery texture. This problem can be prevented by using block-type nonfat cream cheese, and by adding one tablespoon of flour for each cup of nonfat cream cheese used.

Evaporated Skimmed Milk. This ingredient can be substituted for cream in custards, puddings, and other dishes, where it adds creamy richness and nutrients, but no fat.

Milk. Whole milk, the highest-fat milk available, is 3.5 percent fat by weight and has 8 grams of fat per cup. Instead, choose skim (nonfat) milk, which—with all but a trace of fat removed—has only about 0.5 gram of fat per cup. Also a good choice is 1-percent milk, which, as the name implies, is 1 percent fat by weight, and contains 2 grams of fat per cup.

Nonfat Dry Milk. Like evaporated skimmed milk, nonfat dry milk powder adds a creamy richness to custards and puddings while boosting nutritional value. One cup of skim milk mixed with one-third cup of nonfat dry milk powder can replace cream in most recipes. This ingredient may also be added to low-fat, low-sugar cookies and brownies to enhance flavor and browning. Be sure to use *instant* nonfat dry milk powder for the easiest mixing.

Ricotta Cheese. Ricotta is a mild, slightly sweet, creamy cheese that may be used in cheesecakes, frostings, and dessert fillings. As the name implies, nonfat ricotta contains no fat at all. Low-fat and light ricotta, on the other hand, have 1 to 3 grams of fat per ounce, while whole-milk ricotta has 4 grams of fat per ounce.

Soft Curd Farmer Cheese. This soft white cheese makes a good low-fat substitute for cream cheese. Brands made with skim milk have about 3 grams of fat per ounce compared with cream cheese's 10 grams. Soft curd farmer cheese may be used in cheesecakes, frostings, and fillings. Some brands are made with whole milk, so read the label before you buy. Look for a brand like Friendship Farmer Cheese.

Sour Cream. As calorie- and fat-conscious people know, full-fat sour cream can contain almost 500 calories and about 48 grams of fat per cup! Use nonfat sour cream, though, and you'll save 320 calories and 48 grams of fat. Made from cultured nonfat milk thickened with vegetable

gums, this product substitutes beautifully for its fatty counterpart in any dish. In baked goods, plain nonfat yogurt may also be substituted for sour cream.

Yogurt. Yogurt adds creamy richness and flavor to baked goods. In your low-fat cooking, select brands with 1 percent or less milkfat.

Sugar-free flavored nonfat yogurts are especially versatile in diabetic cooking. Try mixing equal parts of vanilla yogurt—or your favorite flavor—with light whipped topping to make a creamy cake frosting or filling. Sugar-free yogurt may also be used in parfaits, puddings, and other desserts that do not require cooking.

Yogurt Cheese. A good substitute for cream cheese in cheesecakes, frostings, and fillings, yogurt cheese can be made at home with any brand of plain or flavored yogurt that does not contain gelatin. Simply place the yogurt in a funnel lined with cheesecloth or a coffee filter, and let it drain into a jar in the refrigerator for eight hours or overnight. When the yogurt is reduced by half, it is ready to use. The whey that collects in the jar may used in place of the liquid in bread and muffin recipes.

Butter, Margarine, Oil, and Fat Substitutes

Most people are surprised to learn that butter, margarine, and oil usually contribute more calories to desserts than sugar does. And sugar-free recipes usually contain as much or more fat than traditional recipes. The reason? It is almost impossible to eliminate both sugar and fat from most dessert recipes and maintain an appealing flavor and consistency. In fact, extra fat may be added to compensate for the loss of texture and taste that occurs when sugar is removed.

Now that some sugar is allowed in diabetic meal plans, fat can be reduced or eliminated in many recipes, and more wholesome desserts—that are still quite low in sugar—can be enjoyed. Many of the recipes in this book do not contain any added fats at all. Instead, fat substitutes like applesauce, fruit purées, fruit juices, buttermilk, and yogurt have been used to moisten baked goods. Some of the recipes in this book also use reduced-fat margarine or light butter instead of their full-fat counterparts. Let's learn a little more about these fat-saving products.

Reduced-Fat Margarine. Contrary to popular belief, you *can* bake with reduced-fat margarine. Replacing regular margarine or butter with a reduced-fat product can cut the fat by as much as 55 percent without greatly affecting taste or texture.

Because reduced-fat products are diluted with water, they cannot be substituted for their full-fat counterparts on a one-for-one basis. If you wish to reduce the fat in your favorite baked goods, replace the desired amount of butter or margarine with three-fourths as much of a reduced-fat brand. For example, if a cookie recipe calls for one cup of margarine, use three-fourths cup of a reduced-fat brand. For best results, use a brand with 5 to 6 grams of fat per tablespoon (full-fat brands contain 10 to 11 grams per tablespoon). Products with less fat than this do not work well in most baked goods.

Light Butter. Like reduced-fat margarine, light butter is diluted with water. This product can replace regular butter in baking using the same guidelines as those used with reduced-fat margarine. When baking, be sure not to confuse whipped butter—butter that has had air whipped into it—with light butter.

Oil. Oil is pure fat—all brands contain 13 grams of fat per tablespoon. For this reason, oil, like other fats, should be used only in small amounts.

Some of the recipes in this book contain a very small amount of oil.

For baking, try unrefined corn oil. Unlike the tasteless refined oils commonly sold in grocery stores, unrefined corn oil has a delicious buttery flavor, and retains much of the corn's nutritional value. Just a little bit adds wonderful flavor to your recipe. Another option for baking is canola oil, which is widely available in grocery stores. Be aware, though, that canola oil will add no flavor to your recipe.

Unrefined oils can be found in health foods stores and some grocery stores. When using these products, keep in mind that they will turn rancid quickly if stored at room temperature. For this reason, it is wise to purchase small bottles (you will not be using much oil anyway). After opening the bottle, store the oil in the refrigerator.

Fat Substitutes. Almost any moist ingredient can replace part or all of the fat in cakes, cookies, brownies, breads, and other baked goods. The recipes in this book use a variety of fat substitutes. All of these substitutes, including applesauce, fruit purées, fruit juices, nonfat buttermilk, and nonfat yogurt, are readily available in most grocery stores.

Egg Whites and Egg Substitutes

Everyone who bakes knows that eggs are indispensable in a wide range of baked goods, from breads to cakes to cookies. Of course, eggs are also loaded with cholesterol and contain some fat as well. For this reason, the recipes in this book call for egg whites or fat-free egg substitute. Just how great are your savings in cholesterol and fat when whole eggs are replaced with one of these ingredients? One large egg contains 80 calories, 5 grams of fat, and 210 milligrams of cholesterol. The equivalent amount of egg white or fat-free egg substitute—3 tablespoons—contains 20 to 30 calories, no fat, and

...erol. The benefits of these substitute ...s are clear.

...ay wonder why some of the recipes in this book call for egg whites while others call for egg substitute. In some cases, one ingredient does, in fact, work better than the other. For instance, egg substitute is the best choice when making puddings and custards. On the other hand, when recipes require whipped egg whites, egg substitutes will not work.

In most recipes, egg whites and egg substitutes can be used interchangeably. Yet, even in these recipes, one may sometimes be listed instead of the other due to ease of measuring. For example, while a cake made with three tablespoons of fat-free egg substitute would turn out just as well if made with three tablespoons of egg whites, this would require you to use one and a half large egg whites, making measuring something of a nuisance.

Whenever a recipe calls for egg whites, use large egg whites. When selecting an egg substitute, look for a fat-free brand like Egg Beaters or Better'n Eggs. (Some egg substitutes contain vegetable oil.) When replacing egg whites with an egg substitute, or whole eggs with egg whites or an egg substitute, use the following guidelines:

1 large egg = $1\frac{1}{2}$ large egg whites
1 large egg = 3 tablespoons egg substitute
1 large egg white = 2 tablespoons egg substitute

Grains and Flours

Just because a food is fat-free or low-fat does not mean it is good for you. Fat-free products made from refined white flour provide few nutrients, and can actually deplete nutrient stores if eaten in excess. Whole grains and whole grain flours, on the other hand, contain a multitude of nutrients such as vitamin E, zinc, magnesium, and chromium—nutrients that can actually help your body better metabolize dietary sugar.

Fortunately, once accustomed to the heartier taste and texture of whole grains, most people prefer them over tasteless refined grains. Following is a description of some whole grain products used in the recipes in this book. Many of these products are readily available in grocery stores, while others may be found in health foods stores and gourmet shops. If you are unable to locate a particular grain or flour in your area, it is probably available by mail order. (See the Resource List on page 153.)

Barley Flour. This flour, made from ground barley kernels, is rich in cholesterol-lowering soluble fiber. Slightly sweet-tasting, barley flour adds a cake-like texture to baked goods, and can be used interchangeably with oat flour in any recipe.

Bread Flour. Designed especially for use in yeast breads, this flour—made of high-gluten wheat flour and dough conditioners—makes yeast doughs rise better.

Brown Rice Flour. Brown rice flour is simply finely ground brown rice. It has a texture similar to that of cornmeal, and adds a mildly sweet flavor to baked goods. Use it in cookies for a crisp and crunchy texture.

Cornmeal. This grain adds a sweet flavor, a lovely golden color, and a crunchy texture to baked goods. Select whole grain (unbolted) cornmeal for the most nutrition. By contrast, bolted cornmeal is nearly whole grain, and degermed cornmeal is refined.

Oat Bran. Made of the outer part of the oat kernel, oat bran has a sweet, mild flavor and is a concentrated source of cholesterol-lowering soluble fiber. Oat bran helps retain moisture in baked goods, making it a natural for fat-free and low-fat baking. Look for it in the hot cereal section of your grocery store, and choose the softer, more finely ground products, like Quaker Oat Bran. Coarsely ground oat bran makes excellent hot cereal, but is not the best choice for most baking purposes.

Oat Flour. This mildly sweet flour is perfect for cakes, muffins, and other baked goods. Like oat bran, oat flour retains moisture in baked goods, and reduces the need for fat. To add extra fiber and nutrients to your own recipes, replace up to one third of the refined wheat flour with oat flour. Available in health foods stores and many grocery stores, oat flour can also be made at home by grinding quick-cooking rolled oats in a blender.

Oats. Loaded with cholesterol-lowering soluble fiber, oats add a chewy texture and sweet flavor to quick breads, cookies, and crumb toppings. They are also delicious in breakfast cereals and other dishes. The recipes in this book use quick-cooking rolled oats. (Look for oats that cook in one minute.)

Unbleached Flour. This is refined white flour that has not been subjected to a bleaching process. Unbleached white flour lacks significant amounts of nutrients compared with whole wheat flour, but does contain more vitamin E than bleached flour.

The unbleached flour that is widely available in supermarkets is a multipurpose flour that can be used in a variety of baked goods recipes, including any recipes in this book that call for unbleached flour. If you can find an *unbleached pastry flour,* it will produce even better results in cakes, pie crusts, cookies, quick breads, and muffin recipes—although you will need to substitute it for regular flour by using the guidelines on page 14. Made from a softer (lower-protein) wheat, unbleached pastry flour will produce a finer, softer texture in baked goods than will regular unbleached flour. Unfortunately, unbleached pastry flour is not widely available. It can, however, be purchased by mail order.

You may have noticed that many fat-free and low-fat recipes include cake flour, which is a finely ground, low-protein flour that is widely available in grocery stores. While cake flour does perform well in baking, it is a highly refined product that has been bleached with chlorine gas. For this reason, cake flour is not used in the recipes in this book.

Whole wheat flour. Made of ground whole grain wheat kernels, whole wheat flour includes the grain's nutrient-rich bran and germ. Nutritionally speaking, whole wheat flour is far superior to refined flour. Sadly, many people grew up eating refined baked goods and find whole grain products too heavy for their taste. A good way to learn to enjoy whole grain flours is to use part whole wheat and part unbleached flour in recipes, and gradually increase the amount of whole wheat used over time.

When cake, cookie, pie crust, quick bread, and other dessert recipes call for whole wheat flour, *whole wheat pastry flour*—also called *whole grain pastry flour*—works best. Whole wheat pastry flour produces lighter, softer-textured baked goods than regular whole wheat flour because it is made from a softer (lower-protein) wheat, and is more finely ground. Whole wheat pastry flour also has a lighter, sweeter flavor than regular whole wheat flour, and so is a natural choice for low-sugar desserts. Look for whole wheat pastry flour in health foods stores and many grocery stores.

White whole wheat flour is another good option when making all your baked goods, including yeast breads. Made from hard white wheat instead of the hard red wheat used to make regular whole wheat flour, white whole wheat flour is sweeter and lighter tasting than its red wheat counterpart. White whole wheat flour is available in many grocery stores and by mail order.

As you can see, there is a wide variety of flours available for use in baking. Experiment with various flours to see which kinds you like best. Here are some guidelines that will allow you to substitute various flours for refined wheat flour in your own favorite recipes:

1 cup refined wheat flour equals:

- ❑ 1 cup unbleached flour
- ❑ 1 cup plus 2 tablespoons unbleached pastry flour
- ❑ 1 cup plus 2 tablespoons cake flour
- ❑ 1 cup whole wheat pastry flour
- ❑ 1 cup minus 1 tablespoon white whole wheat flour
- ❑ 1 cup minus 2 tablespoons regular whole wheat flour
- ❑ 1 cup minus 2 tablespoons brown rice flour
- ❑ 1 cup barley flour
- ❑ 1 cup oat flour

Traditional Caloric Sweeteners

Anyone who has tried to eliminate all of the sugar from a cookie, cake, bread, or muffin recipe knows the value of sugar in baked goods. Sugar adds tenderness and lightness to baked goods and enhances browning during baking. Baked goods made without *any* sugar are tough and coarse-textured, and do not brown properly.

Fortunately, some sugar is now allowable in diabetic diets, making it possible to create truly great desserts that the whole family can enjoy. Just don't get carried away and use gobs of sugar in your desserts! Instead, add as little sugar as you can, use the most healthful ingredients possible, and work your treats into your meal plan instead of having them in addition to your meal plan.

The baked goods and dessert recipes in this book contain 25 to 75 percent less sugar than that used in traditional desserts, and some are totally sugar-free. Ingredients like fruit juices, fruit purées, and dried fruits; flavorings and spices like vanilla extract, nutmeg, and cinnamon; and mildly sweet grains like oats and oat bran have often been used to reduce the need for sugar.

Most of the recipes in this book do call for small amounts of white sugar, brown sugar, or different liquid sweeteners such as honey, molasses, and maple syrup. Do any of these sweeteners offer special advantages to people with diabetes? Not really. All of these sweeteners, as well as the additional caloric sweeteners described below, contain either sucrose—the chemical name for white table sugar—or combinations of glucose and fructose, the two sugars of which sucrose is constituted. All of these sweeteners also raise blood sugar levels similarly. However, some sweeteners, such as honey, are sweeter than sugar, so that less can be used to obtain the desired degree of sweetness. Other sweeteners, like molasses, brown sugar, and date sugar, are more flavorful than white sugar, so that, again, less can be used in many recipes. And some sweeteners, like molasses and date sugar, provide some nutritional value, while refined white sugar provides no nutrients at all. Where do fruit juices fit in? Many of the fruit juice concentrates used for sweetening commercial dessert items are so highly refined that they have been stripped of their vitamins and minerals. All that's left is the sugar. The recipes in this book, though, use *real* fruit juices and juice concentrates—ingredients that retain many of the nutrients of the fruits themselves. Fruit purées are also used, and are even better than juice, since they contain the whole fruit.

A large number of sweeteners are now available, and you should feel free to substitute one for another, using your own tastes, your desire for high-nutrient ingredients, and your pocketbook as a guide. (Some of the newer less-refined sweeteners are far more expensive than traditional sweeteners.) For best results, replace granular sweeteners with other granular sweeteners, and substitute liquid sweeteners for other liquid sweeteners. You can, of course, replace a liquid with granules, or vice versa, but adjustments in other recipe ingredients will have to be made. (For each cup of liquid sweetener substituted for granulated sweetener, reduce the liquid by a fourth to a third of a cup.) Also be aware that each sweetener has its own unique flavor and its own degree of sweetness, making some sweeteners better suited to particular recipes.

Following is a description of some of the sweeteners commonly available in grocery stores, health foods stores, and gourmet shops. Those sweeteners that can't be found in local stores can usually be ordered by mail. (See the Resource List on page 153.)

Apple Butter. Sweet and thick, apple butter is made by cooking down apples with apple juice and spices. Many brands also contain added sugar, but some are sweetened only with apple juice. Use apple butter as you would honey to sweeten products where a little spice will enhance flavor. Spice cakes, bran muffins, and oatmeal cookies are all delicious made with apple butter.

Brown Rice Syrup. Commonly available in health foods stores, brown rice syrup is made by converting the starch in brown rice into sugar. This syrup is mildly sweet—about 30 to 60 percent as sweet as sugar, depending on the brand—and has a delicate malt flavor. This sweetener is not particularly useful in a diabetic diet since, compared with other sweeteners, a relatively large amount has to be used to obtain the desired level of sweetness.

Brown Sugar. This granulated sweetener is simply refined white sugar that has been coated with a thin film of molasses. Light brown sugar is lighter in color than regular brown sugar, but not lower in calories, as the name might imply. Because this sweetener contains some molasses, brown sugar has more calcium, iron, and potassium than white sugar. But like most sugars, brown sugar is no nutritional powerhouse. The advantage to using this sweetener instead of white sugar is that it is more flavorful, so that less can generally be used.

Date Sugar. Made from ground dried dates, date sugar provides copper, magnesium, iron, and B vitamins. With a distinct date flavor, date sugar is delicious in breads, cakes, and muffins. Because it does not dissolve as readily as white sugar does, it's best to mix date sugar with the recipe's liquid ingredients and let it sit for a few minutes before proceeding with the recipe. Less dense than white sugar, this product is only about two-thirds as sweet. However, date sugar is more flavorful, and so can often be substituted for white sugar on a cup-for-cup basis.

Fruit Juice Concentrates. Frozen juice concentrates add sweetness and flavor to baked goods while enhancing nutritional value. Use the concentrates as you would honey or other liquid sweeteners, but beware—too much will be overpowering. Always keep cans of frozen orange and apple juice concentrate in the freezer just for cooking and baking. Pineapple and tropical fruit blends also make good sweeteners, and white grape juice is ideal when you want a more neutral flavor.

Fruit Source. Made from white grape juice and brown rice, this sweetener has a rather neutral flavor and is about as sweet as white sugar. Fruit Source is available in both granular and liquid forms. Use the liquid as you would honey, and the granules as you would sugar. The granules do not dissolve as readily as sugar does, so mix Fruit Source with the recipe's liquid ingredients and let it sit for a few minutes before proceeding with the recipe.

Fruit Spreads, Jams, and Preserves. Available in a variety of flavors, these products make delicious sweeteners. For best flavor and nutrition, choose a brand made from fruits and fruit juice concentrate, with little or no added sugar, and select a flavor that is compatible with the baked goods you're making. Use as you would any liquid sweetener.

Honey. Contrary to popular belief, honey is not significantly more nutritious than sugar, but it does add a nice flavor to baked goods. It also adds moistness, reducing the need for fat. Honey is 20 to 30 percent sweeter than sugar, so less can be used to obtain the desired amount of sweetness.

Maple Sugar. Made from dehydrated maple syrup, granulated maple sugar adds a distinct maple flavor to baked goods. Powdered maple sugar is also available, and can be used to replace powdered white sugar in glazes.

Maple Syrup. The boiled-down sap of sugar maple trees, maple syrup adds a delicious flavor to all baked goods, and also provides some potassium and other nutrients. Use it as you would honey or molasses.

Molasses. Light, or Barbados, molasses is pure sugarcane juice boiled down into a thick syrup. Light molasses provides some calcium, potassium, and iron, and is delicious in spice cakes, muffins, breads, and cookies. Blackstrap molasses is a by-product of the sugar-refining process. Very rich in calcium, potassium, and iron, it has a slightly bitter, strong flavor and is half as sweet as refined sugar. Because of its distinctive taste, more than a few tablespoons in a recipe is overwhelming.

Sucanat. Granules of evaporated sugarcane juice, Sucanat tastes similar to brown sugar. This sweetener provides small amounts of potassium,

chromium, calcium, iron, and vitamins A and C. Use it as you would any other granulated sugar.

Sugarcane Syrup. The process used to make sugarcane syrup is similar to that of making light molasses. Consequently, the syrup has a molasses-like flavor and is nutritionally comparable to the other sweetener.

Throughout our discussion of sweeteners, we have mentioned that some are higher in nutrients than others. Just how much variation is there among sweeteners? The table below compares the amounts of selected nutrients found in one-quarter cup of

Comparing Traditional Sweeteners

Sweetener (¼ cup)	Calories	Calcium (mg)	Iron (mg)	Potassium (mg)
Apple Butter	130	10	0.5	176
Brown Rice Syrup	256	3	0.1	140
Brown Sugar	205	47	1.2	189
Date Sugar	88	10	0.4	209
Fruit Juice Concentrate (apple)	116	14	0.6	315
Fruit Juice Concentrate (orange)	113	23	0.3	479
Fruit Preserves	216	8	0.0	12
Fruit Source (granules)	192	16	0.4	142
Fruit Source (syrup)	176	15	0.4	138
Honey	240	0	0.5	27
Maple Sugar	176	45	0.8	137
Maple Syrup	202	83	1.0	141
Molasses, Blackstrap	170	548	20.2	2,342
Molasses, Light	172	132	4.3	732
Sucanat	142	41	1.6	281
Sugarcane Syrup	210	48	2.9	340
White Sugar	192	1	0	2

different sweeteners. Pay special attention to how the sweeteners compare with white sugar, the most refined of all the sweeteners.

Alternative Caloric Sweeteners

A variety of sweeteners has traditionally been used to replace the sugar in commercially made diabetic and "sugar-free" desserts. Of these, only fructose is available for home baking. However, for people with diabetes, none of these sweeteners really offers any advantages over traditional sweeteners like sugar, honey, and molasses. Below, you will learn the pros and cons of using these sweeteners in baking, and of buying commercial products made with these sweeteners.

Fructose. Made from cornstarch, this granular sweetener looks and tastes like white sugar, and has an equal number of calories. But unlike white sugar, fructose does not require insulin to be utilized by the body, nor does it cause large increases in blood sugar. Fructose is about one and a half times sweeter than sugar, so that less can be used. Despite this, fructose is not recommended in large amounts because it is readily converted to fat, and can raise levels of blood cholesterol and triglycerides. Like white table sugar, fructose is a highly refined sweetener and provides no nutrients. This sweetener is available in most grocery stores, but is very expensive compared with other sweeteners.

Sorbitol, Mannitol, and Xylitol. These sweeteners, which are chemically similar to sugar, are known as sugar alcohols. Sugar alcohols are commonly used in commercially prepared diabetic foods because, like fructose, they do not need insulin to be absorbed, and do not cause large increases in blood sugar. Sugar alcohols are not without problems, though. Eating too much causes gas, bloating, and diarrhea. In addition,

these sweeteners have the same number of calories as does any other sugar. Sugar alcohols are not as sweet as white sugar, so that more must be used to get the same degree of sweetness.

Starch Hydrolysates. These sweeteners, which are used in many commercially made diabetic candies and "sugar-free" sweets, are formed by the breakdown of edible food starches. Starch hydrolysates have almost as many calories as white sugar. Like sugar alcohols, too much of these sweeteners can have a laxative effect.

Artificial Sweeteners

A number of artificial sweeteners are used to replace the sugar in commercially made diabetic and sugar-free desserts. These sweeteners are also widely available for home use. Much of the appeal of these products stems from the fact that they are virtually calorie-free, and are therefore considered a "free food." And, of course, none requires the use of insulin or raises blood sugar levels. However, since these sweeteners lack the bulk and chemical properties of sugar, it is impossible to replace all of the sugar in baked goods like cakes, cookies, breads, and muffins with artificial sweeteners and still get good results. In general, 25 to 30 percent of the sugar in cakes, cookies, breads, muffins, and other baked goods can be replaced with these sweeteners with little noticeable difference in taste or texture. In desserts like puddings, mousses, pies, tarts, and fruit crisps, half or more of the sugar can generally be replaced with an artificial sweetener.

The recipes in this book take advantage of the natural sweetness of fruits, fruit juices, various grains and flours, and flavorings. In most cases, small to moderate amounts of regular sugar are all that is needed for these desserts, so that artificial sweeteners are not required. In some of the recipes, though, artificial sweeteners are used along with sugar to provide a little extra sweetness.

Let's learn about the various artificial sweeteners, and see how you can use them to replace some of the sugar in your own dessert recipes.

Acesulfame-K. Sold under the brand name Sunette and as the table sweeteners Swiss Sweet and Sweet One, acesulfame-K is about 200 times sweeter than sugar, has a pleasant flavor, and leaves no bitter aftertaste. Heat stable, acesulfame-K may be used in cooked desserts.

Aspartame. Originally sold under the brand name NutraSweet and as the table sweetener Equal, aspartame is now also available under many other brand names, including Sweet Thing II and Sweet Mate. This sweetener is made of two amino acids—substances used by the body to build proteins—and, like acesulfame-K, is about 200 times sweeter than sugar. It has a pleasant flavor and leaves no bitter aftertaste.

The aspartame that is available for home use breaks down when exposed to heat, so that it can be added only to cold desserts or to cooked puddings at the end of the cooking time. A specially coated form of aspartame is used in commercial pudding mixes and other foods that require cooking. This heat-stable product is not yet available for home use.

Saccharin. The subject of controversy for many years, saccharin is currently sold with a label warning that its use may cause cancer. A ban on saccharin has been proposed, but is currently being withheld until more evidence becomes available. Heat stable, saccharin may be used for cooking and is 300 times sweeter than sugar. This sweetener does have a bitter aftertaste when included in a recipe in large amounts. The artificial sweeteners Sweet'n Low, Superose, and Sugar Twin all contain saccharin.

Many forms of artificial sweeteners are available, and you should feel free to use your favorite brand, bearing in mind that some brands are not heat stable, and so cannot be used in baked goods. The table on page 19 will enable you to replace some of the sugar in your own recipes with your favorite artificial sweetener.

How safe are artificial sweeteners? The Food and Drug Administration (FDA) has established an Acceptable Daily Intake (ADI) for each sweetener. ADIs are based on the amount of sweetener that a person can consume on a daily basis over a lifetime without experiencing adverse effects. Except in the case of saccharin, the ADIs are dependent on a person's body weight, so that the ADI for smaller people is lower than that for larger people.

The table presented below lists ADIs for each of the major artificial sweeteners. A quick look at the table shows that most people are unlikely to reach their ADI for any of the sweeteners on a daily basis. But a person who relies heavily on these products for sweetening beverages, cereals, and other foods; consumes diet soft drinks; and uses these sweeteners extensively for cooking, could come close. Like all artificial foods, these products should be used only in moderation.

Acceptable Daily Intakes (ADIs) for Artificial Sweeteners

ADI Information	Aspartame	Acesulfame-K	Saccharin
Upper daily limit for a 150-pound person	3,409 mg	1,023 mg	1,000 mg
Milligrams of sweetener per packet	35 mg	50 mg	40 mg
Number of packets to reach ADI for a 150-pound person	97 packets	20 packets	25 packets

Guide to Replacing Sugar With Some Commonly Available Artificial Sweeteners

Amount of White or Brown Sugar	Sugar Substitute Equivalent	Amount of White or Brown Sugar	Sugar Substitute Equivalent
1 teaspoon	$\frac{1}{2}$ packet Equal/Sweet Thing II/ Sweet Mate $\frac{1}{8}$ teaspoon Equal Measure 1 teaspoon Sugar Twin (white or brown) 10 drops Superose Liquid $\frac{1}{2}$ packet Sweet'n Low $\frac{1}{12}$ teaspoon Sweet'n Low Brown $\frac{1}{12}$ teaspoon Sweet'n Low Bulk $\frac{1}{8}$ teaspoon Sweet'n Low Liquid $\frac{1}{2}$ packet Sweet One/Swiss Sweet	$\frac{1}{3}$ cup	8 packets Equal/Sweet Thing II/ Sweet Mate $2\frac{1}{2}$ teaspoons Equal Measure $\frac{1}{3}$ cup Sugar Twin (white or brown) $1\frac{1}{3}$ teaspoons Superose Liquid 8 packets Sweet'n Low $1\frac{1}{4}$ teaspoons Sweet'n Low Brown $1\frac{1}{4}$ teaspoons Sweet'n Low Bulk 2 teaspoons Sweet'n Low Liquid 8 packets Sweet One/Swiss Sweet
2 teaspoons	1 packet Equal/Sweet Thing II/ Sweet Mate $\frac{1}{4}$ teaspoon Equal Measure 2 teaspoons Sugar Twin (white or brown) 20 drops Superose Liquid 1 packet Sweet'n Low $\frac{1}{6}$ teaspoon Sweet'n Low Brown $\frac{1}{6}$ teaspoon Sweet'n Low Bulk $\frac{1}{4}$ teaspoon Sweet'n Low Liquid 1 packet Sweet One/Swiss Sweet	$\frac{1}{2}$ cup	12 packets Equal/Sweet Thing II/ Sweet Mate $3\frac{1}{2}$ teaspoons Equal Measure $\frac{1}{2}$ cup Sugar Twin (white or brown) 2 teaspoons Superose Liquid 12 packets Sweet'n Low 2 teaspoons Sweet'n Low Brown 2 teaspoons Sweet'n Low Bulk 1 tablespoon Sweet'n Low Liquid 12 packets Sweet One/Swiss Sweet
1 tablespoon	$1\frac{1}{2}$ packets Equal/Sweet Thing II/ Sweet Mate $\frac{3}{8}$ teaspoon Equal Measure 1 tablespoon Sugar Twin (white or brown) 30 drops Superose Liquid $1\frac{1}{2}$ packets Sweet'n Low $\frac{1}{4}$ teaspoon Sweet'n Low Brown $\frac{1}{4}$ teaspoon Sweet'n Low Bulk $\frac{1}{2}$ teaspoon Sweet'n Low Liquid $1\frac{1}{2}$ packets Sweet One/Swiss Sweet	$\frac{3}{4}$ cup	18 packets Equal/Sweet Thing II/ Sweet Mate $5\frac{1}{2}$ teaspoons Equal Measure $\frac{3}{4}$ cup Sugar Twin (white or brown) 1 tablespoon Superose liquid 18 packets Sweet'n Low 1 tablespoon Sweet'n Low Brown 1 tablespoon Sweet'n Low Bulk $1\frac{1}{2}$ tablespoons Sweet'n Low Liquid 18 packets Sweet One/Swiss Sweet
$\frac{1}{4}$ cup	6 packets Equal/Sweet Thing II/ Sweet Mate $1\frac{3}{4}$ teaspoons Equal Measure $\frac{1}{4}$ cup Sugar Twin (white or brown) 1 teaspoon Superose Liquid 6 packets Sweet'n Low 1 teaspoon Sweet'n Low Brown 1 teaspoon Sweet'n Low Bulk $1\frac{1}{2}$ teaspoons Sweet'n Low Liquid 6 packets Sweet One/Swiss Sweet	1 cup	24 packets Equal/Sweet Thing II/ Sweet Mate $7\frac{1}{4}$ teaspoons Equal Measure 1 cup Sugar Twin (white or brown) 4 teaspoons Superose Liquid 24 packets Sweet'n Low 4 teaspoons Sweet'n Low Brown 4 teaspoons Sweet'n Low Bulk 2 tablespoons Sweet'n Low Liquid 24 packets Sweet One/Swiss Sweet

Other Ingredients

Aside from the ingredients already discussed, a few more items may prove useful as you venture into low-fat, low-sugar cooking and baking. Some ingredients may already be familiar to you, while others may become new and valuable additions to your pantry.

Barley Nugget Cereal. Crunchy, nutty cereals, like Grape-Nuts nuggets, make a nice addition to crumb toppings, cookies, muffins, and other baked goods whenever you want to reduce or eliminate the use of high-fat nuts.

Dried Fruits. A wide variety of dried fruits are available. Dried pineapple, apricots, prunes, dates, and peaches can be found in most grocery stores, while health foods stores and gourmet shops often carry dried mangoes, papaya, cherries, blueberries, and cranberries. These fruits add interest to muffins, cookies, and other baked goods. If you cannot find the type of dried fruit called for in a recipe, feel free to substitute another type, as all dried fruits contain a similar amount of carbohydrate on a cup-for-cup basis.

Fat-Free Granola. Like barley nugget cereals, fat-free granola is a good substitute for nuts. This product adds a nutty crunch and extra flavor to cookies, breads, and other baked goods. Many low-fat granolas are also available, and are also good options. Look for brands with no more than 2 grams of fat per ounce.

Light Whipped Topping. With half the fat of whipped cream and 40 percent less calories, light whipped toppings like Cool Whip Lite are used in light frostings and fillings, and add creamy richness to mousses and other desserts.

Low-Fat Graham Crackers. Graham crackers have always been fairly low in fat. Now many low-fat and a few fat-free brands are available as well, providing even better choices. The recipes in this book use low-fat graham crackers in both graham cracker pie crusts and crumb toppings.

Low-Sugar Jams and Fruit Spreads. Not to be confused with all-fruit spreads, low-sugar jams and fruit spreads contain about half the sugar of traditional jams and spreads. Some contain artificial sweeteners, and others do not. A low-sugar jam or fruit spread will have about 8 calories per teaspoon, compared with the 16 calories of a full-sugar spread. Some of the recipes in this book call for low-sugar jams, while others use all-fruit spreads.

Nuts. It may surprise you to learn that the recipes in this book sometimes include nuts as an ingredient, or suggest them as an optional addition. True, nuts are high in fat. But when used in small amounts, nuts will not blow your fat budget, and will provide some of the essential fats necessary for good health.

Oat Flake-and-Almond Cereal. Ready-to-eat cereals like Post Honey Bunches of Oats with Almonds, General Mills Oatmeal Crisp with Almonds, and Quaker Toasted Oatmeal With Almonds, can be ground into crumbs just like graham crackers and used to make tasty low-fat pie crusts.

Sugar-Free Gelatin Mixes. Sweetened with aspartame and acesulfame-K, these products are considered a "free food" in diabetic diets. They can be used to make a variety of desserts, including pies, mousses, fruit whips, and parfaits.

Sugar-Free Pudding Mixes. Available in both instant and cook-and-serve varieties, most of the commercial sugar-free pudding mixes are sweetened with acesulfame-K and aspartame. These products may be substituted for the sugar-sweetened mixes used to make your favorite puddings, parfaits, mousses, and pie fillings.

Toasted Wheat Germ. This ingredient adds crunch and nutty flavor to baked goods. A super-nutritious food, with 90 percent less fat than nuts, wheat germ provides generous amounts of vitamin E and minerals.

A Word About Salt

Salt, a combination of sodium and chloride, enhances the flavors of many foods, including baked goods and other desserts. A little salt added to cookie, cake, or other dessert recipes can reduce the need for sugar. For this reason, a few of the recipes in this book list a small amount of salt as an optional ingredient. Dessert breads made with yeast also require some salt, although the amount included in these recipes is about half that used in traditional recipes.

How much sodium is too much? Most health organizations recommend an upper limit of 2,400 milligrams per day, the equivalent of about one teaspoon of salt.

As you probably know, many people with diabetes also have high blood pressure. If you are trying to reduce your blood pressure, you should be aware that sodium is just one of the factors involved in blood pressure regulation. Other nutrients are important as well. Potassium, for instance, works with sodium to control fluid balance in the body. Diets rich in potassium help protect against high blood pressure. Calcium and mag-

nesium are two other minerals that are important for maintaining normal blood pressure. Excess weight can also raise blood pressure. For many people, the loss of just a few pounds can bring their blood pressure under control.

The recipes in this book contain whole grains, fruits, nonfat and low-fat dairy products, and other wholesome ingredients that provide far more potassium, calcium, and magnesium than are supplied by most desserts. In addition, you will find that sodium—as well as fat and calories—is kept under control.

ABOUT THE NUTRITION ANALYSIS

The Food Processor II (ESHA Research) computer nutrition analysis system, along with product information from manufacturers, was used to calculate the nutritional information for the recipes in this book. Dietary exchanges were then calculated based on the amount of carbohydrate, protein, and fat, and the kinds of ingredients included in the recipe.

Diabetic Dream Desserts is full of recipes that can make any meal special, or provide a satisfying between-meals snack. Low in sugar and fat, and high in nutrients, these are wholesome desserts that will fit beautifully into your dietary plan, and that you can feel good about serving to family and friends. Better yet, the dream desserts you are about to make are just that—temptingly sweet treats that are so utterly scrumptious, no one but you will ever guess just how healthy they are!

2

Creative Cakes

If you have ever tried to make a cake without sugar, you understand the importance of this ingredient in baked goods. Besides adding sweetness, sugar inhibits the development of gluten, a protein in flour that can cause cakes to become tough and coarsely textured. That's why so many low- and no-sugar cake recipes call for extra fat. Like sugar, fat keeps gluten from forming.

Fortunately, there are better ways to reduce the sugar in cakes and still maintain a pleasing texture. The secret? Include some healthful whole grain flours in your cake. Whole grain flours are naturally lower in gluten than refined flours. Oat flour and oat bran work especially well in low-sugar, low-fat baked goods. Not only are these products low in gluten, they are also rich in soluble fiber, which helps retain moisture—a boon to the low-fat baker. And since oats have a mildly sweet flavor, they help reduce the need for added sugar. Some of the cakes in this chapter also include whole wheat pastry flour. This versatile product, which has a softer texture and lighter flavor than regular whole wheat flour, will help you make the lightest, most tender cakes possible—

though regular whole wheat flour can be used in many of these recipes with good results, using the guidelines for substitution on page 14.

A number of the recipes in this chapter also feature puréed fruits, applesauce, and fruit juices among the list of ingredients. These healthful additions both moisten and naturally sweeten cake batters, reducing the need for added fat and refined sugar. The result? Super-moist and flavorful cakes that are fat-free or low in fat and contain only moderate amounts of sugar. In fact, most of the sweet treats presented in this chapter contain three to five teaspoons of added sugar per serving. For perspective, a slice of angel food cake or pound cake—the traditionally recommended cake choices for diabetic diets—contains five to six teaspoons of sugar. A slice of iced layer cake can contain as much as twelve teaspoons of sugar!

So whether you are looking for a grand finale to an elegant meal or for a simple coffee cake for a casual get-together, you need look no further. With a little creativity, you and your family will be delighted to find that you *can* have your cake and eat it, too.

Cinnamon Carrot Cake

1. Place the flour, sugar, baking soda, and cinnamon in a large bowl, and stir to mix well. Add the applesauce, egg substitute, carrots, and vanilla extract, and stir to mix well. Stir in the walnuts.

2. Coat a 9-x-13-inch pan with nonstick cooking spray. Spread the batter evenly in the pan, and bake at 325°F for 35 minutes, or just until the top springs back when lightly touched and a wooden toothpick inserted in the center of the cake comes out clean. Allow the cake to cool to room temperature.

3. To make the frosting, place the cream cheese, milk, vanilla extract, and sugar substitute in a medium-sized bowl, and beat with an electric mixer until smooth. Gently fold in the whipped topping.

4. Spread the frosting over the cooled cake. Cut into 2-x-3-inch squares, and serve immediately or refrigerate.

Yield: 18 servings

2 cups unbleached flour

1¼ cups sugar

1½ teaspoons baking soda

1½ teaspoons ground cinnamon

1 cup unsweetened applesauce

¼ cup plus 2 tablespoons fat-free egg substitute

2½ cups (packed) grated carrots (about 5 medium)

2 teaspoons vanilla extract

½ cup chopped walnuts

NUTRITIONAL FACTS (PER SERVING)

Calories: 162 Carbohydrate: 30 g Cholesterol: 1 mg
Fat: 2.8 g Fiber: 1.2 g Protein: 4.9 g Sodium: 187 mg

DIABETIC EXCHANGES: 1 Starch, 1 Fruit, ½ Fat

FLUFFY CREAM CHEESE FROSTING

1 block (8 ounces) nonfat cream cheese

1 tablespoon skim milk

1 teaspoon vanilla extract

Sugar substitute equal to ⅓ cup sugar (page 19)

1½ cups light whipped topping

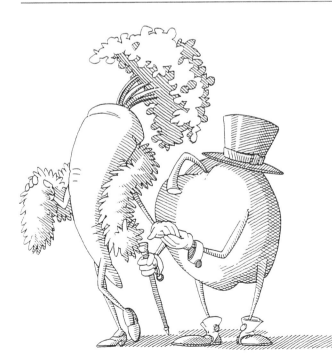

Poppy Seed Pound Cake

Yield: 16 servings

½ cup reduced-fat margarine or light butter, softened to room temperature

1⅓ cups sugar

½ cup fat-free egg substitute

¼ cup plus 1 tablespoon unsweetened applesauce

1½ teaspoons vanilla extract

1 teaspoon lemon or almond extract

1½ cups unbleached flour

½ cup oat bran

1¼ teaspoons baking powder

1 tablespoon poppy seeds

1. Place the margarine or butter and the sugar in the bowl of an electric mixer, and beat to mix well. Add the egg substitute, applesauce, and extracts, and beat to mix well.

2. Place the flour, oat bran, and baking powder in a medium-sized bowl, and stir to mix well. Add the flour mixture to the margarine mixture, and beat just until well mixed. Add the poppy seeds, and beat just until the seeds are mixed in.

3. Coat an 8-x-4-inch loaf pan with nonstick cooking spray, and spread the mixture evenly in the pan. Bake at 350°F for 1 hour, or just until a wooden toothpick inserted in the center of the loaf comes out clean.

4. Remove the cake from the oven, and let sit for 20 minutes. Invert the cake onto a wire rack, turn right side up, and cool to room temperature before slicing and serving.

NUTRITIONAL FACTS (PER SERVING)

Calories: 148   Carbohydrate: 28 g   Cholesterol: 0 mg
Fat: 3.6 g   Fiber: 1 g   Protein: 2.6 g   Sodium: 66 mg

DIABETIC EXCHANGES: 1 Starch, 1 Fruit, ½ Fat

Chocolate Cream Cake Roll

Yield: 12 servings

1⅓ cups unbleached flour

1 cup sugar

⅓ cup cocoa powder

1 teaspoon baking soda

¾ cup unsweetened applesauce

½ cup fat-free egg substitute

¼ cup skim milk

1 teaspoon vanilla extract

1. Place the flour, sugar, cocoa, and baking soda in a medium-sized bowl, and stir to mix well. Add the applesauce, egg substitute, milk, and vanilla extract, and stir to mix well.

2. Line a 15¼-x-10¼-inch jelly roll pan with waxed paper by laying a 16-inch piece of waxed paper in the pan, and folding up the sides so that the paper covers the bottom and sides of the pan. Spray the waxed paper with nonstick cooking spray, and spread the batter evenly in the pan. Bake at 350°F for 12 minutes, or just until the cake springs back when lightly touched. Be careful not to overbake.

3. While the cake is baking, lay a clean kitchen towel out on a work surface. Remove the cake from the oven, and immediately invert it onto the towel. Peel off the waxed paper. Starting at the short end, loosely roll the cake and towel up together. (There should be $1\frac{1}{2}$ inches of open space in the center to accommodate the filling.) Place the cake roll on a wire rack, and allow to cool to room temperature.

4. To make the filling, place the pudding mix and the milk in a small bowl. Whip with a wire whisk for 2 minutes, or until well mixed and thickened. Gently fold in the whipped topping, and set aside.

5. Gently unroll the cooled cake just enough to allow the filling to be spread over the top. Spread the filling to within $\frac{1}{2}$ inch of each edge. Roll the cake up, and transfer to a serving platter. Cover and chill for several hours or overnight.

6. Just before serving, trim $\frac{1}{2}$ inch off each end of the chilled cake, and discard. Slice the cake roll $\frac{3}{4}$ inch thick, and serve.

FILLING

1 package (4-serving size) instant sugar-free chocolate, white chocolate, or pistachio pudding mix

1 cup skim milk

$1\frac{1}{4}$ cups light whipped topping

NUTRITIONAL FACTS (PER SERVING)

Calories: 149 Carbohydrate: 32 g Cholesterol: 0 mg
Fat: 1.4 g Fiber: 1.3 g Protein: 3.6 g Sodium: 244 mg

DIABETIC EXCHANGES: 2 Starch

Cherry Tunnel Cake

1. Place the flour, oat bran, sugar, baking soda, baking powder, and lemon or orange rind in a large bowl, and stir to mix well. Add the buttermilk, oil, egg substitute, and vanilla extract, and stir to mix well.

2. Coat a 12-cup bundt pan with nonstick cooking spray, and spread the batter evenly in the pan. Spoon the cherry filling in a ring over the center of the batter. (The filling will sink into the batter as the cake bakes.)

3. Bake at 350°F for about 40 minutes, or until the top is golden brown and a wooden toothpick inserted on either side of the filling comes out clean. Allow the cake to cool in the pan for 40 minutes. Then invert onto a wire rack, and cool to room temperature.

4. Sift the powdered sugar over the top of the cake just before slicing and serving.

Yield: 20 servings

$2\frac{1}{4}$ cups unbleached flour

$\frac{3}{4}$ cup oat bran

$1\frac{1}{3}$ cups sugar

1 teaspoon baking soda

1 teaspoon baking powder

1 teaspoon dried grated lemon or orange rind

$1\frac{1}{4}$ cups nonfat or low-fat buttermilk

3 tablespoons vegetable oil

$\frac{1}{4}$ cup plus 1 tablespoon fat-free egg substitute

$1\frac{1}{2}$ teaspoons vanilla extract

$1\frac{1}{3}$ cups light (reduced-sugar) cherry pie filling

2 tablespoons powdered sugar

NUTRITIONAL FACTS (PER SERVING)

Calories: 152 Carbohydrate: 30 g Cholesterol: 0 mg
Fat: 2.5 g Fiber: 1.2 g Protein: 3 g Sodium: 105 mg

DIABETIC EXCHANGES: 1 Starch, 1 Fruit, $\frac{1}{2}$ Fat

Angel Pudding Cake

Yield: 12 servings

2 cups skim milk

1 package (4-serving size) instant or cook-and-serve sugar-free white or dark chocolate pudding mix

3 cups sliced fresh strawberries

1½ cups fresh raspberries

1 angel food cake (1 pound)

FROSTING

1 cup plus 2 tablespoons light whipped topping

1/4 cup plus 2 tablespoons sugar-free nonfat vanilla, strawberry, or raspberry yogurt

1. Use the skim milk to prepare the pudding according to package directions. Chill the pudding for at least 1 hour, or until thickened.

2. Place the strawberries and raspberries in a large bowl, tossing to mix well. Set aside.

3. Using a serrated knife, cut a 1½-inch-deep channel in the top of the cake, leaving ⅜ inch of the cake intact on either side of the channel. Place the cake in the center of a 12-inch round platter. Spoon the chilled pudding evenly into the hollowed-out section of the cake. Arrange 1½ cups of the fruit mixture over the pudding. (The fruit will mound slightly over the top.)

4. To make the frosting, place the whipped topping in a small bowl, and gently fold the yogurt into the topping. Spread the mixture over the sides and top of the cake so that the frosting meets the edges of the fruit. Arrange the remaining fruit around the base of the cake. Chill for 2 hours before slicing and serving.

NUTRITIONAL FACTS (PER SERVING)

Calories: 145 Carbohydrates: 31 g Cholesterol: 1 mg
Fat: 1.2 g Fiber: 1.3 g Protein: 3.8 g Sodium: 388 mg

DIABETIC EXCHANGES: 1 Starch, 1 Fruit

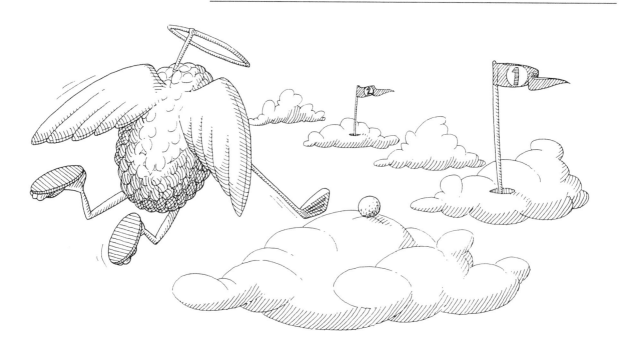

Fudge Cake With Raspberry Sauce

1. To make the raspberry sauce, place the cornstarch in a 1-quart saucepan, and stir in first the juice, and then the raspberries. Heat the mixture to boiling over medium heat, stirring constantly. Cook for about 3 minutes, still stirring, until the raspberries break up and the mixture is thick and bubbly.

2. Remove the pot from the heat, and allow to cool for 5 minutes. Stir the sugar substitute into the raspberry mixture. Transfer to a covered container, and refrigerate until ready to serve.

3. Place the flours, sugar, cocoa, baking soda, and salt in a large bowl, and stir with a wire whisk to mix well. Add the water, sour cream, and vanilla extract, and stir to mix well.

4. Coat a 9-inch round baking pan with nonstick cooking spray, and spread the batter evenly in the pan. Bake at 350°F for about 18 minutes, or just until the top springs back when lightly touched and a wooden toothpick inserted in the center of the cake comes out clean. Be careful not to overbake. Allow the cake to cool to room temperature.

5. When ready to serve, cut the cake into 8 wedges and top each serving with 2 tablespoons of the chilled sauce.

Yield: 8 servings

$\frac{2}{3}$ cup unbleached flour

$\frac{1}{3}$ cup oat flour

$\frac{1}{2}$ cup plus 2 tablespoons sugar

$\frac{1}{4}$ cup cocoa powder

$\frac{3}{4}$ teaspoon baking soda

$\frac{1}{4}$ teaspoon salt

$\frac{1}{2}$ cup plus 2 tablespoons water

$\frac{1}{3}$ cup nonfat sour cream

1 teaspoon vanilla extract

RASPBERRY SAUCE

1 tablespoon cornstarch

$\frac{1}{4}$ cup white grape juice

$1\frac{1}{2}$ cups fresh or frozen (unthawed) raspberries

Sugar substitute equal to $\frac{1}{4}$ cup sugar (page 19)

NUTRITIONAL FACTS (PER SERVING)

Calories: 150   Carbohydrate: 32 g   Cholesterol: 0 mg
Fat: 1 g   Fiber: 2.2 g   Protein: 3 g   Sodium: 199 mg

DIABETIC EXCHANGES: 1 Starch, 1 Fruit

FAT-FIGHTING TIP

Chocolate Flavor With a Fraction of the Fat

For rich chocolate flavor with minimal fat, substitute cocoa powder for high-fat baking chocolate. Simply use three tablespoons of cocoa powder plus one tablespoon of water or another liquid to replace each ounce of baking chocolate in cakes, brownies, puddings, and other goodies. You'll save 111 calories and 13.5 grams of fat for each ounce of baking chocolate you replace!

For the deepest, darkest, richest cocoa flavor, use Dutch processed cocoa in your chocolate treats. Dutching, a process that neutralizes the natural acidity in cocoa, results in a darker, sweeter, more mellow-flavored cocoa. Look for a brand like Hershey's Dutch Processed European Style cocoa. Like regular cocoa, this product has only a half gram of fat per tablespoon. (Beware, though, as some brands contain more fat.) Dutched cocoa can be substituted for regular cocoa in any recipe. And since Dutched cocoa has a smoother, sweeter flavor, you may find that you can reduce the sugar in your recipe by up to 25 percent.

Mocha Fudge Cake

Yield: 18 servings

1¼ cups unbleached flour

¾ cup oat flour

1 cup plus 2 tablespoons sugar

¼ cup plus 2 tablespoons cocoa
powder

1½ teaspoons baking soda

½ teaspoon salt

1 cup skim milk

¾ cup plus 1 tablespoon coffee,
cooled to room temperature

1 tablespoon distilled white
vinegar

1½ teaspoons vanilla extract

½ cup chopped walnuts

GLAZE

1 cup powdered sugar

2 tablespoons cocoa powder

1 tablespoon plus 2 teaspoons
coffee, cooled to room
temperature

1½ teaspoons vanilla extract

1. Place the flours, sugar, cocoa, baking soda, and salt in a large bowl, and stir with a wire whisk to mix well.

2. Place the milk, coffee, vinegar, and vanilla extract in a small bowl, and stir to mix well. Add the milk mixture to the flour mixture, and stir with a wire whisk until the batter is smooth. (The batter will be thin.) Stir in the walnuts.

3. Coat a 9-x-13-inch pan with nonstick cooking spray, and pour the batter into the pan. Bake at 350°F for 30 minutes, or just until the top springs back when lightly touched and a wooden toothpick inserted in the center of the cake comes out clean. Be careful not to overbake.

4. To make the glaze, place all of the glaze ingredients in a small bowl, and stir until smooth. Spread the glaze in a thin layer over the hot cake. Allow the cake to cool to room temperature in the pan, and cut into 2-x-3-inch squares to serve.

NUTRITIONAL FACTS (PER SERVING)

Calories: 145   Carbohydrate: 29 g   Cholesterol: 0 mg
Fat: 2.7 g   Fiber: 1.8 g   Protein: 2.9 g   Sodium: 165 mg

DIABETIC EXCHANGES: 2 Starch, ½ Fat

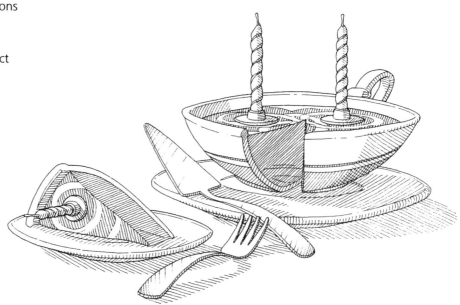

Chocolate-Almond Cannoli Cake

This cake is made in a flan or tiara pan. The bottom of the pan has a raised center that makes an ideal place to put the filling after the cake has been baked, cooled, and inverted.

1. Place the flours, sugar, cocoa, baking soda, and salt in a medium-sized bowl, and stir with a wire whisk to mix well.

2. Place the water, vinegar, and extracts in a small bowl, and stir to mix well. Add the water mixture to the flour mixture, and stir with a wire whisk to mix well. (The batter will be thin.)

3. Coat a 10-inch flan pan with nonstick cooking spray, and pour the batter into the pan. Bake at 350°F for 15 minutes, or just until the top springs back when lightly touched and a wooden toothpick inserted in the center of the cake comes out clean. Be careful not to overbake.

4. Allow the cake to cool to room temperature in the pan. Then invert the cake onto a serving platter.

5. To make the filling, place the ricotta, sugar, sugar substitute, and vanilla extract in a food processor, and process until smooth. Fill the depression in the top of cake with the filling. Sprinkle the almonds over the filling, and chill for several hours before slicing and serving.

Yield: 10 servings

¾ cup unbleached flour

¾ cup oat flour

¾ cup sugar

¼ cup cocoa powder

1 teaspoon baking soda

⅛ teaspoon salt

1¼ cups water

1½ teaspoons distilled white vinegar

1 teaspoon vanilla extract

½ teaspoon almond extract

FILLING

15 ounces nonfat ricotta cheese

2 tablespoons sugar

Sugar substitute equal to ⅓ cup sugar (page 19)

¾ teaspoon vanilla extract

¼ cup sliced toasted almonds (page 87)

NUTRITIONAL FACTS (PER SERVING)

Calories: 183 Carbohydrate: 34 g Cholesterol: 6 mg
Fat: 1.9 g Fiber: 1.9 g Protein: 9 g Sodium: 211 mg

DIABETIC EXCHANGES: 2 Starch, ½ Skim Milk

Golden Pear Cake

Yield: 9 servings

¾ cup unbleached flour

½ cup whole wheat pastry flour

½ cup light brown sugar

¾ teaspoon baking soda

⅛ teaspoon ground cardamom

½ cup plain nonfat yogurt

2 egg whites, lightly beaten

2 cups chopped peeled fresh
   pears (about 2½ medium)

¼ cup golden raisins

TOPPING

1 tablespoon light brown sugar

1 tablespoon toasted wheat germ

1. To make the topping, place the brown sugar and wheat germ in a small bowl, and stir to mix well. Set aside.

2. Place the flours, brown sugar, baking soda, and cardamom in a medium-sized bowl, and stir to mix well. Add the yogurt and egg whites, and stir just until well mixed. Fold in the pears and raisins.

3. Coat an 8-inch square pan with cooking spray. Spread the batter in the pan, and sprinkle with the topping. Bake at 350°F for 30 to 35 minutes, or just until a toothpick inserted in the center of the cake comes out clean and the top springs back when lightly touched.

4. Allow the cake to cool for at least 30 minutes before cutting into squares and serving. Serve warm or at room temperature.

NUTRITIONAL FACTS (PER SERVING)

Calories: 144   Carbohydrate: 32 g   Cholesterol: 0 mg
Fat: 0.5 g   Fiber: 2.3 g   Protein: 4 g   Sodium: 132 mg

DIABETIC EXCHANGES: 1 Starch, 1 Fruit

German Chocolate Delight

Yield: 10 servings

¾ cup unbleached flour

¾ cup oat flour

¾ cup light brown sugar

¼ cup cocoa powder

1 teaspoon baking soda

⅛ teaspoon salt

1¼ cups water

1½ teaspoons distilled white
   vinegar

1 teaspoon vanilla extract

½ teaspoon coconut-flavored
   extract

Like the Chocolate-Almond Cannoli Cake (page 31), this cake is made in a flan or tiara pan, allowing you to add a "filling" after the cake has been baked and cooled.

1. Place the flours, brown sugar, cocoa, baking soda, and salt in a medium-sized bowl, and stir with a wire whisk to mix well.

2. Place the water, vinegar, and extracts in a small bowl, and stir to mix well. Add the water mixture to the flour mixture, and stir with a wire whisk to mix well. (The batter will be thin.)

3. Coat a 10-inch flan pan with nonstick cooking spray, and pour the batter into the pan. Bake at 350°F for 15 minutes, or just until the top springs back when lightly touched and a wooden toothpick inserted in the center of the cake comes out clean. Be careful not to overbake.

4. Allow the cake to cool to room temperature in the pan. Then invert the cake onto a serving platter.

5. To make the filling, combine the pudding mix and milk in a small bowl. Stir with a wire whisk for 2 minutes, or until well mixed and thickened. Fold in the coconut and pecans. Fill the depression in the top of cake with the filling, and chill for several hours before slicing and serving.

FILLING

1 package (4-serving size) instant sugar-free butterscotch pudding mix

1½ cups skim milk

⅓ cup shredded sweetened coconut

⅓ cup chopped pecans

NUTRITIONAL FACTS (PER SERVING)

Calories: 177 Carbohydrate: 32 g Cholesterol: 0 mg
Fat: 4.2 g Fiber: 2 g Protein: 4.2 g Sodium: 264 mg

DIABETIC EXCHANGES: 2 Starch, 1 Fat

Peachy Kuchen Cake

1. To make the topping, place the almonds, sugar, and cinnamon in a small bowl, and stir to mix well. Set aside.

2. Place the flours, sugar, baking powder, and baking soda in a medium-sized bowl, and stir to mix well. Add the yogurt, egg substitute, and vanilla extract, and stir just until well mixed. (The batter will be fairly thick.)

3. Coat a 10-inch round cake pan with nonstick cooking spray, and spread the batter over the bottom of the pan. Arrange the peach slices in concentric circles over the top of the cake; then scatter the blueberries over the peaches. Sprinkle the topping over the batter and fruit.

4. Bake at 350°F for about 35 minutes, or just until a wooden toothpick inserted in the center of the cake comes out clean and the top springs back when lightly touched. (Choose a spot that contains no fruit.)

5. Allow the cake to cool for at least 30 minutes before cutting into wedges and serving. Serve warm or at room temperature.

Yield: 10 servings

¾ cup unbleached flour

½ cup whole wheat pastry flour

¾ cup sugar

1½ teaspoons baking powder

¼ teaspoon baking soda

¼ cup plus 2 tablespoons plain nonfat yogurt

¼ cup fat-free egg substitute

1½ teaspoons vanilla extract

1 can (1 pound) sliced peaches in juice, well drained

1 cup fresh or frozen (unthawed) blueberries

TOPPING

2 tablespoons finely ground almonds

1 tablespoon sugar

¼ teaspoon ground cinnamon

NUTRITIONAL FACTS (PER SERVING)

Calories: 151 Carbohydrate: 32 g Cholesterol: 0 mg
Fat: 1.1 g Fiber: 2.1 g Protein: 3 g Sodium: 97 mg

DIABETIC EXCHANGES: 1 Starch, 1 Fruit

Light and Luscious Lemon Cake

Yield: 16 servings

For variety, substitute other flavors of gelatin and yogurt for the lemon.

1 box (1 pound, 2.25 ounces) light (reduced-fat) white cake mix, prepared

2 packages (4-serving size each) sugar-free lemon gelatin mix

1 cup boiling water

1 cup cool tap water

FROSTING

1$\frac{1}{2}$ cups light whipped topping

1 cup sugar-free nonfat lemon yogurt

1. Prepare the cake according to package directions, baking it in a 9-x-13-inch pan. Allow the cake to cool to room temperature. Then, using a fork, poke holes in the cake at $\frac{1}{2}$-inch intervals.

2. Place the gelatin mix in a medium-sized bowl. Pour the boiling water over the gelatin, and stir until dissolved. Stir in the cool water. Slowly pour the gelatin mixture over the cake, allowing it to be absorbed. Cover and refrigerate for at least 3 hours.

3. To make the frosting, place the whipped topping in a small bowl, and gently fold in the yogurt. Spread the frosting over the cake, and chill for an additional hour before cutting into squares and serving.

NUTRITIONAL FACTS (PER SERVING)

Calories: 154 Carbohydrate: 30 g Cholesterol: 0 mg
Fat: 3 g Fiber: 0.3 g Protein: 2.8 g Sodium: 264 mg

DIABETIC EXCHANGES: 2 Starch, $\frac{1}{2}$ Fat

Cranberry-Orange Coffee Cake

Yield: 20 servings

$\frac{1}{2}$ cup reduced-fat margarine or light butter, softened to room temperature

1$\frac{1}{4}$ cups sugar

4 egg whites, or $\frac{1}{2}$ cup fat-free egg substitute

1$\frac{1}{2}$ teaspoons vanilla extract

1 cup nonfat buttermilk

2$\frac{1}{4}$ cups unbleached flour

$\frac{3}{4}$ cup oat bran

2 teaspoons baking powder

$\frac{1}{2}$ teaspoon baking soda

1 tsp dried grated orange rind

1. Place the margarine or butter and the sugar in the bowl of an electric mixer, and beat until smooth. Beat in the egg whites and vanilla extract. Beat in the buttermilk.

2. Place the flour, oat bran, baking powder, baking soda, and orange rind in a medium-sized bowl, and stir to mix well. Add the flour mixture to the margarine mixture, and beat just until well mixed.

3. To make the filling, transfer $\frac{3}{4}$ cup of the batter to a small bowl. Add the cranberries, sugar substitute, and nuts, and stir to mix.

4. Coat a 12-cup bundt pan with nonstick cooking spray, and spread two-thirds of the plain batter evenly in the pan. Spoon the cranberry batter in a ring over the center of the plain batter, and top with the remaining plain batter.

5. Bake at 350°F for 35 to 40 minutes, or just until a wooden toothpick inserted in the center of the cake comes out clean. Allow the cake to cool in the pan for 30 minutes. Then invert onto a wire rack and cool to room temperature.

6. To make the glaze, combine the powdered sugar, orange rind, and orange juice in a small bowl, and stir until smooth. Transfer the cake to a serving platter, and drizzle the glaze over the cake. Let the cake sit for at least 15 minutes, allowing the glaze to harden, before slicing and serving.

NUTRITIONAL FACTS (PER SERVING)

Calories: 150 Carbohydrate: 29 g Cholesterol: 0 mg
Fat: 3.2 g Fiber: 1.2 g Protein: 3.2 g Sodium: 111 mg

DIABETIC EXCHANGES: 1 Starch, 1 Fruit, ½ Fat

FILLING

¾ cup whole fresh or frozen (unthawed) cranberries, finely chopped

Sugar substitute equal to ¼ cup sugar (page 19)

3 tablespoons finely chopped pecans

GLAZE

⅓ cup powdered sugar

½ teaspoon dried grated orange rind

2 teaspoons orange juice

Sour Cream Apple Coffee Cake

1. To make the topping, place the brown sugar and walnuts in a small bowl, and stir to mix well. Set aside.

2. Place the flours, sugar, baking soda, and cinnamon in a medium-sized bowl, and stir to mix well. Stir in the apple juice, sour cream, and egg white. Fold in the apples and walnuts.

3. Coat a 9-inch round pan with nonstick cooking spray. Spread the batter evenly in the pan, and sprinkle with the topping. Bake at 350°F for 30 minutes, or just until a wooden toothpick inserted in the center of the cake comes out clean and the top springs back when lightly touched.

4. Allow the cake to cool for at least 30 minutes before cutting into wedges and serving. Serve warm or at room temperature.

NUTRITIONAL FACTS (PER SERVING)

Calories: 165 Carbohydrate: 32 g Cholesterol: 0 mg
Fat: 2.9 g Fiber: 1.9 g Protein: 3.8 g Sodium: 140 mg

DIABETIC EXCHANGES: 1 Starch, 1 Fruit, ½ Fat

Yield: 10 servings

1 cup unbleached flour

½ cup whole wheat pastry flour

½ cup sugar

1 teaspoon baking soda

1 teaspoon ground cinnamon

½ cup apple juice

¼ cup nonfat sour cream

1 egg white, lightly beaten

2½ cups thinly sliced peeled apples (about 3 medium)

¼ cup chopped walnuts

TOPPING

2 tablespoons light brown sugar

2 tablespoons finely chopped walnuts

Blueberry Bundt Cake

Yield: 20 servings

1/2 cup reduced-fat margarine or light butter, softened to room temperature

1 1/3 cups sugar

1/4 cup plus 2 tablespoons fat-free egg substitute, or 3 egg whites

2 teaspoons vanilla extract

2 1/2 cups unbleached flour

1/2 cup oat bran

1 tablespoon baking powder

1 teaspoon dried grated lemon or orange rind

3/4 cup skim milk

2 cups fresh or frozen (unthawed) blueberries

GLAZE

1/3 cup powdered sugar

2 teaspoons skim milk

1/4 teaspoon vanilla extract

1. Place the margarine or butter and the sugar in the bowl of an electric mixer, and beat to mix well. Add the egg substitute and vanilla extract, and beat to mix well.

2. Place the flour, oat bran, baking powder, and lemon or orange rind in a medium-sized bowl, and stir to mix well. Add a third of the flour mixture and a third of the skim milk to the margarine mixture, and beat to mix well. Repeat this procedure until all of the flour and milk has been mixed in.

3. Coat a 12-cup bundt pan with nonstick cooking spray, and spread half of the batter evenly in the pan. Sprinkle with 1 cup of the berries, and gently press the berries into the batter. Spoon the remaining batter over the berries, and sprinkle the remaining cup of berries over the batter, again pressing the berries into the batter.

4. Bake at 350°F for about 50 minutes, or just until a wooden toothpick inserted in the center of the cake comes out clean. Allow the cake to cool in the pan for 30 minutes. Then invert the cake onto a wire rack, and cool to room temperature.

5. To make the glaze, place the powdered sugar, milk, and vanilla extract in a small bowl, and stir to mix well. Transfer the cake to a serving platter, and spoon the glaze over the cake. Let the cake sit for at least 15 minutes, allowing the glaze to harden, before slicing and serving.

NUTRITIONAL FACTS (PER SERVING)

Calories: 154   Carbohydrate: 31 g   Cholesterol: 0 mg
Fat: 2.8 g   Fiber: 1.3 g   Protein: 2.9 g   Sodium: 88 mg

DIABETIC EXCHANGES: 1 Starch, 1 Fruit, 1/2 Fat

Mini Cherry Cheesecakes

1. Line 12 muffin cups with paper muffin liners, and spray the liners with nonstick cooking spray. Place 1 vanilla wafer, flat side down, in the bottom of each cup. Set aside.

2. To make the cheese filling, place the cream cheese, ricotta, and sugar in the bowl of a food processor, and process until well mixed. Add the sugar substitute, egg substitute, flour, vanilla extract, and lemon rind, and process until smooth.

3. Divide the filling among the muffin cups, spooning it over the wafers. Bake at 325°F for 30 minutes, or until the cheesecakes are puffed and the filling is set. Turn the oven off, and allow the cheesecakes to cool in the oven for 30 minutes with the door ajar.

4. Refrigerate the cheesecakes, leaving them in the muffin tins, for at least 4 hours. Top each serving with a slightly rounded tablespoon of pie filling just before serving.

Yield: 12 servings

12 reduced-fat vanilla wafers

1 cup light (reduced-sugar) cherry pie filling

CHEESE FILLING

2 blocks (8 ounces each) nonfat cream cheese

1 cup nonfat ricotta cheese

½ cup sugar

Sugar substitute equal to ½ cup sugar (page 19)

½ cup fat-free egg substitute

3 tablespoons unbleached flour

1½ teaspoons vanilla extract

1 teaspoon dried grated lemon rind

NUTRITIONAL FACTS (PER SERVING)

Calories: 126   Carbohydrate: 21 g   Cholesterol: 3 mg
Fat: 0.4 g   Fiber: 0.2 g   Protein: 10 g   Sodium: 245 mg

DIABETIC EXCHANGES: 1 Starch, ½ Skim Milk

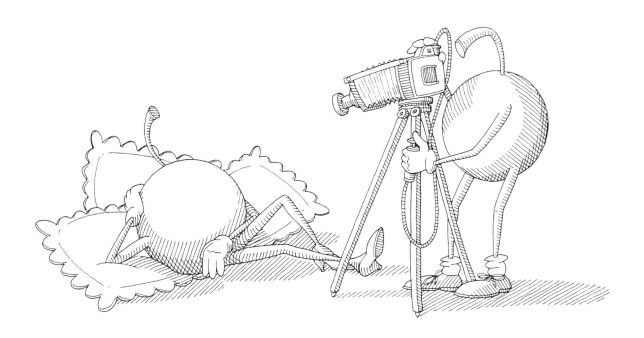

Cocoa-Zucchini Snack Cake

Yield: 9 servings

¾ cup unbleached flour

¼ cup plus 2 tablespoons whole wheat pastry flour

⅔ cup sugar

3 tablespoons cocoa powder

1 teaspoon baking powder

¼ teaspoon baking soda

⅛ teaspoon salt

¾ teaspoon ground cinnamon

½ cup nonfat or low-fat buttermilk

2 egg whites, lightly beaten

1 teaspoon vanilla extract

1 cup finely grated unpeeled zucchini (about 1 medium)

¼ cup dark raisins

¼ cup chopped walnuts

1. Place the flours, sugar, cocoa, baking powder, baking soda, salt, and cinnamon in a medium-sized bowl, and stir to mix well. Add the buttermilk, egg whites, and vanilla extract, and stir just enough to mix well. Stir in first the zucchini, and then the raisins and walnuts.

2. Coat an 8-inch square pan with nonstick cooking spray, and spread the mixture evenly in the pan. Bake at 325°F for 30 minutes, or just until a wooden toothpick inserted in the center of the cake comes out clean and the top springs back when lightly touched.

3. Allow the cake to cool to room temperature before cutting into squares and serving.

NUTRITIONAL FACTS (PER SERVING)

Calories: 157 Carbohydrate: 31 g Cholesterol: 0 mg
Fat: 2.4 g Fiber: 1.7 g Protein: 3.9 g Sodium: 132 mg

DIABETIC EXCHANGES: 1 Starch, 1 Fruit, ½ Fat

Fudge Marble Cheesecake

Yield: 10 servings

CRUST

5 large (2½-x-5-inch) reduced-fat chocolate graham crackers

2 tablespoons finely chopped walnuts

1 tablespoon sugar

1 tablespoon fat-free egg substitute

1. To make the crust, break the crackers into pieces, and place in the bowl of a food processor. Process into fine crumbs. Measure the crumbs. There should be ¾ cup. (Adjust the amount if necessary.)

2. Return the crumbs to the food processor, add the walnuts and sugar, and process for a few seconds to mix. Add the egg substitute, and process until the mixture is moist and crumbly.

3. Coat a 9-inch springform pan with nonstick cooking spray, and use the back of a spoon to press the mixture against the bottom and ¼ inch up the sides of the pan, forming an even crust. (Dip the spoon in sugar periodically, if necessary, to prevent sticking.) Bake at 350°F for 8 minutes, or until the edges feel firm and dry. Set aside to cool.

4. To make the cheese filling, place the cream cheese, ricotta, and sugar in the bowl of a food processor, and process until well mixed. Add the sugar substitute, egg substitute, flour, and vanilla extract, and process until smooth. Set aside.

5. To make the fudge filling, transfer $\frac{1}{2}$ cup of the cheese filling to a small bowl. Add the cocoa, sugar, sugar substitute, and vanilla extract, and stir to mix well. Set aside.

6. Spread half of the plain cheesecake batter evenly over the crust. Spoon the fudge filling randomly over the batter; then top with the remaining batter. Draw a knife through the batter to produce a marbled effect.

7. Bake at 325°F for 1 hour, or until the center is set. Turn the oven off, and allow the cake to cool in the oven with the door ajar for 30 minutes.

8. Refrigerate the cake for at least 8 hours. Remove the collar of the pan just before slicing and serving.

NUTRITIONAL FACTS (PER SERVING)
Calories: 197 Carbohydrate: 28 g Cholesterol: 4 mg
Fat: 2 g Fiber: 0.9 g Protein: 15 g Sodium: 350 mg

DIABETIC EXCHANGES: 1 Starch, 1 Skim Milk, $\frac{1}{2}$ Fat

CHEESE FILLING

2 blocks (8 ounces each) nonfat cream cheese, softened to room temperature

15 ounces nonfat ricotta cheese

$\frac{1}{2}$ cup sugar

Sugar substitute equal to $\frac{1}{2}$ cup sugar (page 19)

$\frac{1}{2}$ cup fat-free egg substitute

$\frac{1}{4}$ cup plus 1 tablespoon unbleached flour

2 teaspoons vanilla extract

FUDGE FILLING

3 tablespoons Dutch processed cocoa powder

2 tablespoons sugar

Sugar substitute equal to 2 tablespoons sugar (page 19)

$\frac{3}{4}$ teaspoon vanilla extract

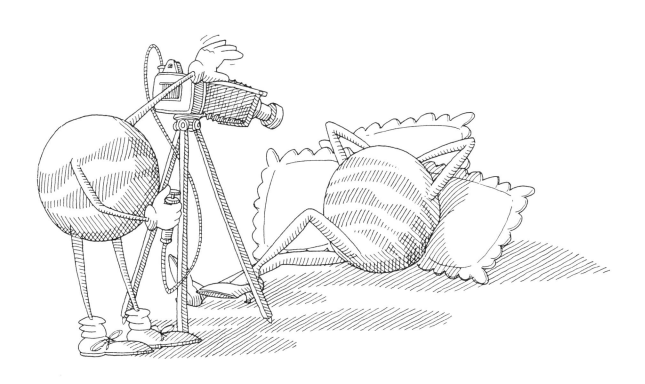

The Icing on the Cake

Traditionally, recipes for icing 9-x-13-inch cakes have often called for up to 3 cups of powdered sugar and a stick of butter. But is there an alternative that not only is healthy, but also satisfies everyone's expectations of a sweet and creamy topping? Of course there is! Instead of being laden with fat, the icings and frostings in this book are made with nonfat ricotta cheese, nonfat cream cheese, light whipped topping, and nonfat yogurt. Just as important, they contain only a fraction of the sugar found in traditional recipes.

The following suggestions summarize many of the icings, frostings, and other no-bake toppings used within these pages, and present some other ideas as well.

❑   Dust the tops of chocolate cakes with a bit of powdered sugar. Try sifting powdered maple sugar over the tops of spice cakes, banana cakes, and other fruit-flavored cakes.

❑   Combine 2 cups of nonfat ricotta cheese, 1 teaspoon of vanilla extract, and 3 to 4 tablespoons of honey or maple syrup in a blender or food processor, and process until smooth. Spread over spice cakes, banana cakes, and other fruit-flavored cakes. This makes enough for a 9-x-13-inch cake.

❑   Instead of using a frosting, spread a thin layer of low-sugar fruit spread or preserves over the tops of cakes. Try raspberry spread on chocolate cakes, pineapple spread on banana cakes, and apricot or peach spread on spice cakes.

❑   Spread cakes with yogurt cheese—a sweet, creamy spread made by draining the whey from yogurt. (See page 10.) To cover a 9-x-13-inch cake, use 2 cups of yogurt cheese, which is made with 4 cups of yogurt. Try vanilla, coffee, or raspberry yogurt cheese on chocolate cakes; vanilla, banana, or pineapple yogurt cheese on banana cakes; and lemon or vanilla yogurt cheese on lemon and carrot cakes.

❑   For a light and fluffy cream cheese icing, combine 8 ounces of nonfat or reduced-fat cream cheese, sugar substitute equal to $\frac{1}{3}$ cup sugar, 1 tablespoon milk, and 1 teaspoon vanilla extract in a bowl, and beat with an electric mixer until smooth. Then fold $1\frac{1}{2}$ cups of light whipped topping into the cheese mixture. Spread over carrot cakes, pineapple cakes, and spice cakes. This makes enough for a 9-x-13-inch cake.

❑   For a fluffy, no-fuss whipped cream-type frosting, fold $\frac{1}{2}$ to 1 cup of sugar-free nonfat yogurt (any flavor) into $1\frac{1}{2}$ cups of light whipped topping. This will frost a 9-x-13-inch cake. Use vanilla yogurt on cakes of any flavor, lemon yogurt on lemon cakes, banana yogurt on banana cakes, and coffee or raspberry yogurt on chocolate cakes. Adding yogurt to whipped toppings creates a creamier flavor and texture, and adds some nutrition to an otherwise nutrient-poor product.

❑   For a super-creamy and deliciously sweet frosting, combine one 4-serving size package (any flavor) of instant sugar-free pudding with 1 cup of skim or low-fat milk. Whip with a wire whisk for 2 minutes, or until smooth and thickened. Then fold in 1 to $1\frac{1}{2}$ cups of light whipped topping. This recipe is practically sugar-free and makes enough frosting for a 9-x-13-inch sheet cake or an 8- or 9-inch double-layer cake. Try chocolate or pistachio flavors on chocolate cakes, butterscotch or banana flavors on spice cakes, and lemon or vanilla flavors on white cakes, lemon cakes, and carrot cakes.

3

Pleasing Pies, Tarts, and Pastries

Flaky and delicious, pies, tarts, and pastries are always a welcome treat. And whether made with a juicy fruit filling or a creamy custard filling, these goodies can easily be prepared with very little sugar and fat. Believe it or not, pies, tarts, and pastries can also add a respectable amount of nutrition to your meal. For example, a low-fat, low-sugar fruit pie with an oatmeal crust will provide some of the fruit and starch exchanges in your meal.

If you compare the recipes in this chapter with those in traditional cookbooks, you will see that they have 50 to 75 percent less sugar than most comparable recipes. The fruit desserts in this chapter get much of their sweetness from fresh fruit, dried fruit, and fruit juices. Spices like cinnamon and nutmeg, as well as flavorings like vanilla extract, have been added to enhance the natural sweetness of these ingredients. For the very best results, always use ripe, sweet fruit. Then you will not need to add a lot of extra sugar.

Like the fruit desserts, the pudding and custard treats in this chapter are low in sugar com-

pared with traditionally prepared confections. Most of these recipes use a combination of sugar and artificial sweeteners to provide a pleasing amount of sweetness without a sugar overload. Some also use commercial sugar-free pudding and gelatin mixes—great time-saving ingredients to have on hand for your low-sugar pie- and tart-making adventures.

What about pie crusts? Most traditional crusts are loaded with fatty shortenings. Even worse, they can be a real ordeal to make from scratch. Not these. As you will see, low-fat, low-sugar crumb crusts prepared with graham crackers or other wholesome ingredients are a snap to make. Even rolled pie crusts can be made with a minimum of fuss, and with less than half the fat of a traditional crust.

So take out your pie and tart pans, and get ready to enjoy a galaxy of homemade goodies. Lusciously sweet and meltingly tender, these are desserts that you will find yourself making time and time again.

PIE CRUSTS

Flaky Oat Pie Crust

This pie crust has half the fat of most traditional crusts, with a light, tender, flaky texture. Fill it with either precooked fillings or fillings that require baking.

Yield: One 9-inch pie crust

$\frac{1}{2}$ cup quick-cooking oats

$\frac{2}{3}$ cup unbleached flour

$\frac{3}{4}$ teaspoon baking powder

$\frac{1}{8}$ teaspoon salt

2 tablespoons vegetable oil

3 tablespoons skim milk

1. Place the oats, flour, baking powder, and salt in a medium-sized bowl, and stir to mix. Add the oil and just enough of the milk to form a stiff dough, stirring just until the mixture holds together and forms a ball.

2. Coat two 12-x-12-inch pieces of waxed paper with nonstick cooking spray. Lay the dough on 1 of the sheets of waxed paper, and pat it into a 7-inch circle. Place the other sheet of waxed paper over the circle of dough, and, using a rolling pin, roll the dough into an 11-inch circle.

3. Coat a 9-inch pie pan with nonstick cooking spray. Peel the top sheet of waxed paper from the pie crust. With the bottom sheet of waxed paper still adhering to the crust, invert the crust over the pie pan. Carefully peel the waxed paper from the crust, and press the crust into the pie pan. Pinch the edges of the crust or press with the tines of a fork to make a decorative edge.

4. For a prebaked crust, prick the crust with a fork at 1-inch intervals, and bake at 400°F for about 12 minutes, or until lightly browned and crisp. Allow the crust to cool to room temperature before filling. When a prebaked crust is not desired, simply fill and bake the crust as directed in the recipe.

NUTRITIONAL FACTS (PER $\frac{1}{8}$ CRUST)

Calories: 89 Carbohydrate: 11.6 g Cholesterol: 0 mg
Fat: 3.8 g Fiber: 1 g Protein: 2 g Sodium: 69 mg

DIABETIC EXCHANGES: $\frac{3}{4}$ Starch, $\frac{3}{4}$ Fat

Crunchy Nutty Pie Crust

Yield: One 9-inch pie crust

1 cup barley nugget cereal

¼ cup finely chopped pecans

2 tablespoons light brown sugar

3 tablespoons fat-free egg substitute

You can fill this scrumptious crust with either precooked fillings or fillings that require baking.

1. Place the cereal, pecans, and brown sugar in a small bowl, and stir to mix well. Stir in the egg substitute.

2. Coat a 9-inch pie pan with nonstick cooking spray, and use the back of a spoon to press the mixture against the bottom and sides of the pan, forming an even crust.

3. Bake the pie shell at 350°F for 12 minutes, or until the edges feel firm and dry. Cool the crust to room temperature and fill with a precooked filling, or fill and bake as directed in the recipe. (Note that this crust should be prebaked even when making pies that require additional baking, such as pumpkin and sweet potato pies. When further baking is required, cut 3-inch-wide strips of aluminum foil, and fold them over the edges of the pie pan to prevent overbrowning.)

NUTRITIONAL FACTS (PER ⅛ CRUST)

Calories: 80   Carbohydrate: 14 g   Cholesterol: 0 mg
Fat: 2 g   Fiber: 1.5 g   Protein: 2.4 g   Sodium: 105 mg

DIABETIC EXCHANGES: 1 Starch, ½ Fat

Lite Graham Cracker Pie Crust

Yield: One 9-inch pie crust

8½ large (2½-x-5-inch) low-fat plain or chocolate graham crackers

Sugar substitute equal to 2 tablespoons sugar (page 19)

2 tablespoons fat-free egg substitute, or 1 large egg white

Fill this crust only with precooked or no-cook fillings, such as puddings.

1. Break the crackers into pieces, and place in the bowl of a food processor. Process into fine crumbs. Measure the crumbs. There should be 1⅓ cups. (Adjust the amount if necessary.)

2. Return the crumbs to the food processor, and add the sugar substitute. Process for a few seconds to mix well. Add the egg substitute or egg white, and process to mix well. The mixture should be moist and crumbly, and should hold together when pinched. If the mixture seems too sticky, add more graham cracker crumbs.

3. Coat a 9-inch pie pan with nonstick cooking spray, and use the back of a spoon to press the mixture against the sides and bottom of the pan, forming an even crust. If necessary, periodically dip the back of the spoon in sugar to prevent sticking.

4. Bake the pie shell at 350°F for 10 to 12 minutes, or until the edges feel firm and dry. Allow the crust to cool to room temperature before filling.

NUTRITIONAL FACTS (PER $\frac{1}{8}$ CRUST)

Calories: 75 Carbohydrate: 15 g Cholesterol: 0 mg
Fat: 0.9 g Fiber: 0.6 g Protein: 1.5 g Sodium: 133 mg

DIABETIC EXCHANGES: 1 Starch

Coconut-Oat Pie Crust

Like the Lite Graham Cracker Pie Crust (page 44), this crust should be filled only with precooked or no-cook fillings.

Yield: One 9-inch pie crust

2$\frac{1}{4}$ cups oat flake-and-almond cereal

$\frac{1}{4}$ cup shredded sweetened coconut

2 tablespoons fat-free egg substitute

$\frac{1}{2}$ teaspoon coconut-flavored extract

1. Place the cereal in the bowl of a food processor, and process into fine crumbs. Measure the crumbs. There should be 1$\frac{1}{8}$ cups. (Adjust the amount if necessary.)

2. Return the crumbs to the food processor, and add the coconut. Process for about 20 seconds, or until the coconut is finely shredded and the mixture is well blended. Add the egg substitute and extract, and process until the mixture is moist and crumbly.

3. Coat a 9-inch pie pan with nonstick cooking spray, and use the back of a spoon to pat the mixture evenly against the sides and bottom of the pan, forming an even crust. If necessary, periodically dip the spoon in sugar to prevent sticking.

4. Bake the pie shell at 350°F for about 12 minutes, or until the edges are golden brown. Allow the crust to cool to room temperature before filling.

NUTRITIONAL FACTS (PER $\frac{1}{8}$ CRUST)

Calories: 77 Carbohydrate: 13 g Cholesterol: 0 mg
Fat: 2.2 g Fiber: 1.1 g Protein: 1.9 g Sodium: 62 mg

DIABETIC EXCHANGES: 1 Starch, $\frac{1}{2}$ Fat

PIES, TARTS, & PASTRIES

Old-Fashioned Pumpkin Pie

Yield: 8 servings

1 unbaked Flaky Oat Pie Crust
  (page 43)

FILLING

1 can (1 pound) pumpkin

1¼ cups evaporated skimmed
  milk

½ cup fat-free egg substitute

¼ cup plus 2 tablespoons light
  brown sugar

Brown sugar substitute equal to
  ¼ cup plus 2 tablespoons
  brown sugar (page 19)

1 teaspoon ground cinnamon*

½ teaspoon ground nutmeg*

½ teaspoon ground ginger*

¼ teaspoon ground cloves*

1½ teaspoons vanilla extract

*If desired, use 2¼ teaspoons of
pumpkin pie spice in place of the
four spices.

1. To make the filling, place all of the filling ingredients in a blender
or food processor, and blend until smooth. Pour the filling into the
prepared crust.

2. Bake at 400°F for 15 minutes. Reduce the heat to 350°F and bake
for 45 additional minutes, or until a sharp knife inserted in the center
of the pie comes out clean. Cover the pie loosely with aluminum foil
during the last 10 minutes of baking if the crust starts to brown too
quickly.

3. Allow the pie to cool to room temperature before cutting into
wedges and serving. Refrigerate any leftovers.

NUTRITIONAL FACTS (PER SERVING)

Calories: 175   Carbohydrate: 28 g   Cholesterol: 1 mg
Fat: 4 g   Fiber: 2.5 g   Protein: 7 g   Sodium: 150 mg

DIABETIC EXCHANGES: 1½ Starch, ½ Skim Milk, ¾ Fat

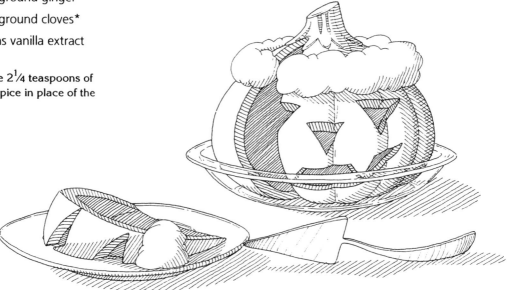

Apple Crumb Pie

For variety, substitute peaches or pears for the apples.

Yield: 8 servings

1. To make the topping, place the cereal, flour, brown sugar, and cinnamon in a small bowl, and stir to mix well. Add the juice concentrate, and stir until the mixture is moist and crumbly. Set aside.

2. To make the filling, place the sugar, cornstarch, and cinnamon in a 4-quart pot, and stir to mix well. Stir in the apple juice.

3. Place the pot over medium-low heat and bring to a boil, stirring constantly. Add the apples and raisins, and stir for a minute or 2, or until the fruit is coated with a thick glaze. Remove the pot from the heat, and stir in the sugar substitute.

4. Spread the filling evenly in the crust, and sprinkle the topping over the filling. Bake at 400°F for 15 minutes. Reduce the heat to 375°F and bake for 30 to 35 additional minutes, or until the filling is bubbly around the edges and the topping is golden brown. Cover the pie loosely with aluminum foil during the last 10 minutes of baking if the topping starts to brown too quickly.

5. Allow the pie to cool for at least 30 minutes before cutting into wedges and serving. Serve warm or at room temperature.

1 unbaked Flaky Oat Pie Crust (page 43)

FILLING

2 tablespoons sugar

1 tablespoon plus 1½ teaspoons cornstarch

½ teaspoon ground cinnamon

¼ cup plus 1 tablespoon unsweetened apple juice

6 cups sliced peeled apples (6 to 8 medium)

¼ cup dark raisins

Sugar substitute equal to ¼ cup sugar (page 19)

TOPPING

¼ cup barley nugget cereal

3 tablespoons whole wheat pastry flour

3 tablespoons light brown sugar

½ teaspoon ground cinnamon

1 tablespoon frozen apple juice concentrate, thawed

NUTRITIONAL FACTS (PER SERVING)

Calories: 208 Carbohydrate: 40 g Cholesterol: 0 mg
Fat: 4 g Fiber: 3.4 g Protein: 3.1 g Sodium: 112 mg

DIABETIC EXCHANGES: 1 Starch, 1½ Fruit, 1 Fat

DREAM DESSERT TIP

Pie Apples That Please

Dozens of varieties of apples are available in grocery stores. Many of the crisp, sweet varieties that we love to eat out of hand, however, can become mushy when cooked. For best results when making pies, crisps, and tarts, use a firm-textured variety such as Crispin, Fuji, Golden Delicious, Granny Smith, Jonathan, Newton Pippin, Rome, or Winesap. The sweetest of these varieties—Crispin, Fuji, Golden Delicious, and Rome—will require the least amount of added sugar.

Pear Phyllo Pie

Yield: 8 servings

CRUST

2 tablespoons sugar

1/2 teaspoon ground cinnamon

1/4 teaspoon ground nutmeg

6 sheets (14 x 18 inches) phyllo pastry (about 5 ounces)

Butter-flavored cooking spray

FILLING

2 tablespoons sugar

Sugar substitute equal to 3 tablespoons sugar (page 19)

1 tablespoon plus 1 1/2 teaspoons cornstarch

1/4 teaspoon ground cinnamon

1/4 teaspoon ground nutmeg

6 cups sliced peeled pears (about 6 medium)

2 tablespoons dried currants or chopped dark raisins

1. To make the filling, place the sugar, sugar substitute, cornstarch, cinnamon, and nutmeg in a small bowl. Stir to mix well.

2. Place the pears in a large bowl. Sprinkle the sugar mixture over the pears, and toss to mix well. Toss in the currants or raisins, and set aside.

3. To make the crust, combine the sugar, cinnamon, and nutmeg in a small dish, and stir to mix well. Set aside.

4. Spread the phyllo dough out on a clean dry surface. Cover the dough with plastic wrap to prevent it from drying out as you work. (Remove sheets as you need them, being sure to re-cover the remaining dough.)

5. Remove 1 sheet of phyllo dough, and lay it on a clean dry surface. Spray the dough lightly with the cooking spray, and sprinkle with 1 teaspoon of the sugar mixture. Top with another phyllo sheet, spray with cooking spray, and sprinkle with the sugar mixture.

6. Coat a 9-inch pie pan with nonstick cooking spray, and gently press the double-stacked phyllo sheets into the pan, allowing the ends to extend over the edges. Rotate the pie pan slightly, and repeat the procedure with 2 more sheets. Rotate the pan again, and repeat with the 2 remaining sheets.

7. Spread the filling evenly in the crust, and fold the phyllo in to cover the filling. Spray the top lightly with nonstick cooking spray, and sprinkle the remaining sugar mixture over the top. Using a sharp knife, score through the top crust to make 8 wedges. (This will prevent the crust from flaking excessively when the pie is cut into serving pieces.)

8. Bake at 350°F for 40 to 45 minutes, or until the top is golden brown. Allow to cool for at least 30 minutes before cutting into wedges and serving. Serve warm or at room temperature.

NUTRITIONAL FACTS (PER SERVING)
Calories: 157   Carbohydrate: 33 g   Cholesterol: 0 mg
Fat: 1.4 g   Fiber: 3.3 g   Protein: 1.6 g   Sodium: 69 mg

DIABETIC EXCHANGES: 1 Starch, 1 Fruit, 1/3 Fat

Making Pear Phyllo Pie.

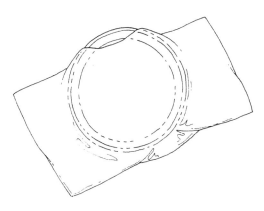

a. Press 1 set of phyllo sheets into the pan.

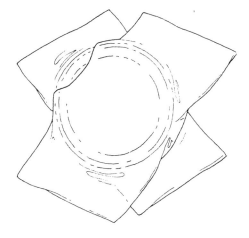

b. Rotate the pan, and press in another set of sheets.

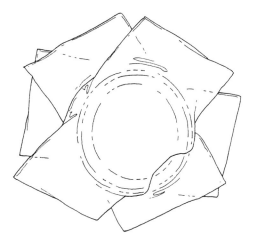

c. Rotate the pan, and press in the remaining sheets.

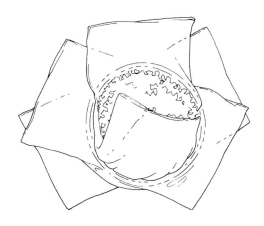

d. Fold the pastry over the filling.

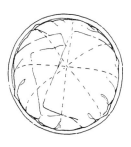

e. Score the pastry to make 8 wedges.

Southern Sweet Potato Pie

Yield: 8 servings

1 prebaked Crunchy Nutty Pie
    Crust (page 44)

FILLING

1 pound sweet potatoes (about 2
    medium)

1 cup evaporated skimmed milk

$\frac{1}{2}$ cup fat-free egg substitute

$\frac{1}{4}$ cup dark brown sugar

Brown sugar substitute equal to
    $\frac{1}{3}$ cup brown sugar (page 19)

2 teaspoons ground cinnamon

$\frac{1}{2}$ teaspoon ground nutmeg

1 teaspoon vanilla extract

1.   If using a conventional oven, bake the potatoes at 400°F for about 45 minutes, or until tender. If using a microwave oven, prick the potatoes with a fork at 1-inch intervals and bake at high power for 12 minutes, or until tender. Set the potatoes aside to cool. Then peel and cut into 1-inch pieces.

2.   Place the potatoes and all of the remaining filling ingredients in a blender or food processor, and blend until smooth. Pour the filling into the prepared crust. Cut 3-inch-wide strips of aluminum foil, and fold over the edges of the pie pan to shield the crust.

3.   Bake at 350°F for 50 minutes, or until a sharp knife inserted in the center of the pie comes out clean. Allow to cool to room temperature before cutting into wedges and serving. Refrigerate any leftovers.

NUTRITIONAL FACTS (PER SERVING)

Calories: 178   Carbohydrate: 31 g   Cholesterol: 1 mg
Fat: 2.7 g   Fiber: 2.5 g   Protein: 7 g   Sodium: 165 mg

DIABETIC EXCHANGES: 2 Starch, $\frac{1}{4}$ Skim Milk, $\frac{1}{2}$ Fat

---

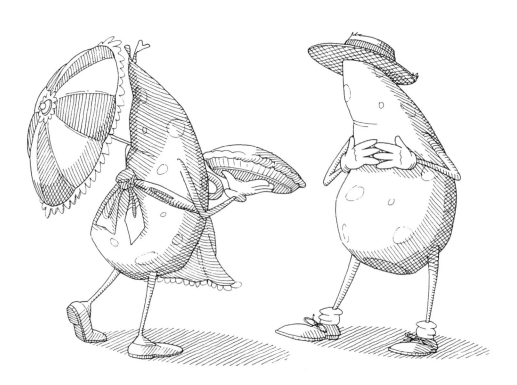

Fabulous Fruit Pie

1. To make the glaze, place the cornstarch and sugar in a 1½-quart pot, and stir to mix well. Slowly stir in first the orange juice, and then the crushed pineapple with all of the juice. Cook and stir over medium-low heat until the mixture is thickened and bubbly. Set aside to cool for 15 minutes.

2. Spread half of the pineapple mixture evenly over the bottom of the prepared crust. Arrange the strawberries in a circular pattern over the pineapple mixture. Arrange the kiwi slices over the strawberries. Arrange the banana slices over the kiwi. Top with the remaining pineapple mixture, and garnish with the strawberry slices.

3. Chill the pie for several hours, or until the glaze is set, before cutting into wedges and serving. Serve chilled.

Yield: 8 servings

1 prebaked Coconut-Oat Pie Crust (page 45) or Crunchy Nutty Pie Crust (page 44)

FILLING

1 cup sliced fresh strawberries

2 kiwi fruit, peeled and sliced ¼ inch thick

1 cup sliced bananas

5 strawberry slices (garnish)

GLAZE

2 tablespoons plus 1½ teaspoons cornstarch

2 tablespoons sugar

¾ cup orange juice

1 can (8 ounces) crushed pineapple in juice, undrained

NUTRITIONAL FACTS (PER SERVING)

Calories: 157 Carbohydrate: 32 g Cholesterol: 0 mg
Fat: 2.4 g Fiber: 2.5 g Protein: 1.9 g Sodium: 25 mg

DIABETIC EXCHANGES: 1 Starch, 1 Fruit, ½ Fat

Banana Dream Pie

1. To make the filling, use the skim milk to prepare the pudding according to package directions. Remove the pudding from the heat and allow to cool for 5 minutes, stirring twice.

2. Spoon a third of the pudding over the bottom of the pie crust. Top with the bananas, and spoon the remaining pudding over the bananas.

3. Chill the pie for several hours, or until the filling is set. When ready to serve, top each slice with a rounded tablespoon of whipped topping. Serve chilled.

Yield: 8 servings

1 prebaked Lite Graham Cracker Pie Crust made with plain or chocolate graham crackers (page 44) or Coconut-Oat Pie Crust (page 45)

FILLING

2¾ cups skim milk

1 package (6-serving size) cook-and-serve sugar-free vanilla pudding mix

2 cups bananas, sliced ¼ inch thick (about 2½ medium)

TOPPING

¾ cup light whipped topping

NUTRITIONAL FACTS (PER SERVING)

Calories: 152 Carbohydrate: 30 g Cholesterol: 1 mg
Fat: 1.7 g Fiber: 1.2 g Protein: 4.5 g Sodium: 233 mg

DIABETIC EXCHANGES: 1 Starch, 1 Fruit, ¼ Skim Milk

Mocha Mousse Pie

Yield: 8 servings

1 prebaked Lite Graham Cracker
　Pie Crust made with chocolate
　graham crackers (page 44)

FILLING

¼ cup plus 2 tablespoons skim
　milk

1 envelope unflavored gelatin

15 ounces nonfat ricotta cheese

¼ cup sugar

¼ cup cocoa powder

2 teaspoons instant coffee
　granules

Sugar substitute equal to ½ cup
　sugar (page 19)

2 teaspoons vanilla extract

1 cup light whipped topping

TOPPING

½ cup light whipped topping

Cocoa powder

1. To make the filling, place the milk in a 1-quart pot. Sprinkle the gelatin over the milk, and let sit for 2 minutes to allow the gelatin to soften. After 2 minutes, place over low heat and cook and stir for about 3 minutes, or until the gelatin is completely dissolved. (Do not let the mixture boil.) Transfer the mixture to a medium-sized mixing bowl, and set aside for about 20 minutes to cool to room temperature.

2. Place the ricotta, sugar, cocoa, coffee granules, sugar substitute, and vanilla extract in a food processor, and process until smooth. Set aside.

3. When the gelatin mixture has reached room temperature, beat at high speed with an electric mixer for about 2 minutes, or until the mixture resembles soft whipped cream. Add the ricotta mixture, and beat just long enough to mix well. Gently fold in the whipped topping.

4. Spoon the mixture into the pie shell, mounding the top slightly. Chill the pie for several hours, or until firm. When ready to serve, top each slice with a tablespoon of light whipped topping and a sprinkling of cocoa. Serve chilled.

NUTRITIONAL FACTS (PER SERVING)

Calories: 169　Carbohydrate: 26 g　Cholesterol: 9 mg
Fat: 3.4 g　Fiber: 1.1 g　Protein: 10.9 g　Sodium: 187 mg

DIABETIC EXCHANGES: 1 Starch, 1 Skim Milk, ½ Fat

Raspberry Bavarian Pie

Yield: 8 servings

1 prebaked Lite Graham Cracker
　Pie Crust made with plain or
　chocolate graham crackers
　(page 44)

1. Place the gelatin mix in a small heatproof bowl, and pour the boiling water over the mix. Stir until the gelatin is completely dissolved. Chill the mixture for about 25 minutes, or until it is very thick but not yet solid.

2. Place the ricotta, 2 tablespoons of the sugar, and the vanilla extract in a food processor, and process until smooth. Set aside, leaving the mixture in the processor.

3. Place the raspberries and the remaining tablespoon of sugar in a small bowl, and mash with a fork. Set aside.

4. Add the cooled gelatin mixture to the ricotta mixture, and process just until well mixed. Transfer the ricotta mixture to a large bowl, and gently fold in first the raspberries, and then the whipped topping.

5. Spoon the mixture into the pie shell, mounding the top slightly. Chill the pie for several hours, or until firm, before cutting into wedges and serving. Serve chilled.

FILLING

1 package (4-serving size) sugar-free raspberry gelatin mix

$\frac{1}{2}$ cup boiling water

$1\frac{1}{2}$ cups nonfat ricotta cheese

3 tablespoons sugar, divided

1 teaspoon vanilla extract

1 cup fresh or frozen (thawed) raspberries

$1\frac{1}{2}$ cups light whipped topping

NUTRITIONAL FACTS (PER SERVING)

Calories: 169 Carbohydrate: 28 g Cholesterol: 4 mg
Fat: 2.4 g Fiber: 1.2 g Protein: 9 g Sodium: 173 mg

DIABETIC EXCHANGES: 1 Starch, 1 Milk, $\frac{1}{2}$ Fat

Sensational Strawberry Pie

1. To make the glaze, place the cornstarch and sugar in a 1-quart pot, and stir to mix well. Stir in the juice, and bring to a boil over medium heat, stirring constantly. Reduce the heat to low, and cook and stir for an additional minute, or until the mixture is thickened and bubbly.

2. Remove the pot from the heat, and sprinkle the gelatin over the juice mixture. Using a wire whisk, whisk in first the gelatin, and then the sugar substitute. Set the mixture aside for 20 minutes.

3. To make the filling, place the berries in a large bowl. Stir the glaze, and pour over the berries, tossing gently to coat. Spread the strawberry mixture evenly in the prepared crust.

4. Chill the pie for several hours, or until the glaze is set, before cutting into wedges and serving. Serve chilled.

Yield: 8 servings

1 prebaked Crunchy Nutty Pie Crust (page 44) or Lite Graham Cracker Pie Crust made with plain or chocolate graham crackers (page 44)

FILLING

4 cups halved fresh strawberries

GLAZE

3 tablespoons cornstarch

2 tablespoons sugar

$1\frac{1}{2}$ cups cranberry-strawberry juice (or another strawberry juice blend)

$1\frac{1}{2}$ teaspoons unflavored gelatin

Sugar substitute equal to $\frac{1}{3}$ cup sugar (page 19)

NUTRITIONAL FACTS (PER SERVING)

Calories: 152 Carbohydrate: 31 g Cholesterol: 0 mg
Fat: 2.4 g Fiber: 2.7 g Protein: 2.8 g Sodium: 107 mg

DIABETIC EXCHANGES: 1 Starch, 1 Fruit, $\frac{1}{2}$ Fat

Good – doesn't hold up well – but tasty

Apricot Custard Tart

Yield: 8 servings

1 prebaked Lite Graham Cracker Pie Crust made with plain or chocolate graham crackers (page 44)*

FILLING

1¾ cups skim milk

1 package (4-serving size) instant sugar-free vanilla pudding mix

TOPPING

1 can (1 pound) apricot halves in juice, undrained

2 tablespoons sugar

1 tablespoon cornstarch

*When making the crust, press the mixture over the bottom and 1 inch up the sides of a 9-inch tart or springform pan.

1. To make the filling, pour the milk into a medium-sized bowl. Add the pudding mix, and beat with a wire whisk or electric mixer for 2 minutes, or until the mixture starts to thicken. Immediately pour the pudding into the cooled shell and refrigerate for at least 10 minutes, or until the pudding starts to set.

2. Drain the apricot halves well, reserving the juice and 1 of the apricot halves. Arrange the remaining apricot halves, cut side down, on top of the pudding.

3. Place ½ cup of the reserved apricot juice, the reserved apricot half, the sugar, and the cornstarch in a blender or food processor, and blend until smooth. Pour the mixture into a small saucepan, place over medium heat, and cook, stirring constantly, until the mixture is thickened and bubbly. Allow to cool for 5 minutes. Then stir the mixture and drizzle it over the top of the tart, covering the apricot halves.

4. Refrigerate the tart for several hours, or until set, before cutting into wedges and serving.

NUTRITIONAL FACTS (PER SLICE)
Calories: 147 Carbohydrate: 30 g Cholesterol: 1 mg
Fat: 1 g Fiber: 1.3 g Protein: 4 g Sodium: 227 mg

DIABETIC EXCHANGES: 1 Starch, 1 Fruit

Phyllo Fruit Tarts

Yield: 6 servings

CRUSTS

1 tablespoon plus 1 teaspoon sugar

¼ teaspoon dried grated lemon rind

4 sheets (14 x 18 inches) phyllo pastry (about 3½ ounces)

Butter-flavored cooking spray

1. To make the crusts, combine the sugar and lemon rind in a small dish, and stir to mix well. Set aside.

2. Spread the phyllo dough out on a clean dry surface. Cover the dough with plastic wrap to prevent it from drying out as you work. (Remove sheets as you need them, being sure to re-cover the remaining dough.)

3. Remove 1 sheet of phyllo dough, and lay it on a clean dry surface. Spray the dough lightly with the cooking spray, and sprinkle with 1 teaspoon of the sugar mixture. Top with another phyllo sheet, spray with cooking spray, and sprinkle with the sugar mixture. Repeat with the 2 remaining sheets.

4. Cut the stack of phyllo sheets lengthwise into two 18-inch-long strips. Then cut each strip crosswise to make 3 pieces, each approximately 6 x 7 inches. You should now have 6 stacks of phyllo squares, each 4 layers thick.

5. Coat six jumbo muffin cups or six 6-ounce custard cups with nonstick spray. Gently press 1 stack of phyllo squares into each cup, pleating as necessary, to make it fit. Press the corners back slightly.

6. Bake at 350°F for about 8 minutes, or until golden brown. Remove the crusts from the oven and allow to cool for 5 minutes. Transfer the crusts to wire racks to cool completely. (Note that the crusts may be prepared the day before you plan to serve the tarts, and stored in an airtight container until ready to use.)

7. To prepare the filling, place the cream cheese, ricotta, sugar, and vanilla extract in a food processor, and process until smooth. Spoon 3 tablespoons of the cheese mixture into each crust, and top with $\frac{1}{3}$ cup of sliced strawberries.

8. Place the fruit spread or jam and the juice in a small saucepan, and stir to mix. Cook over medium-low heat, stirring constantly, just until heated through. Drizzle 2 teaspoons of the jam mixture over the strawberries in each tart, and serve immediately.

FILLING

$\frac{3}{4}$ cup nonfat cream cheese

$\frac{1}{2}$ cup nonfat ricotta cheese

2 tablespoons sugar

$\frac{1}{2}$ teaspoon vanilla extract

2 cups sliced fresh strawberries

2 tablespoons strawberry fruit spread or jam

2 tablespoons cranberry or white grape juice

NUTRITIONAL FACTS (PER SERVING)

Calories: 192   Carbohydrate: 35 g   Cholesterol: 1 mg
Fat: 1.4 g   Fiber: 0.9 g   Protein: 8.3 g   Sodium: 228 mg

DIABETIC EXCHANGES: 1 Starch, 1 Fruit, $\frac{1}{2}$ Milk

Making Phyllo Fruit Tarts.

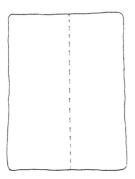

a. Cut the phyllo sheets into 2 long strips.

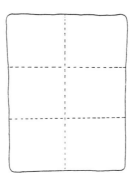

b. Cut each strip crosswise to make 3 squares.

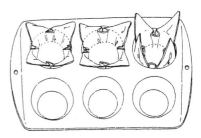

c. Press 1 stack of squares into each muffin cup.

Maple Pear Pie

Yield: 8 servings

1 unbaked Flaky Oat Pie Crust
(page 43)

FILLING

6 cups sliced peeled pears (about
6 medium-large)

Brown sugar substitute equal to
$^1/_3$ cup brown sugar (page 19)

1 tablespoon plus 1 teaspoon
cornstarch

$^3/_4$ teaspoon ground cinnamon

$^1/_4$ teaspoon ground nutmeg

SYRUP

2 teaspoons cornstarch

$^1/_4$ cup plus 1 tablespoon
unsweetened apple juice

3 tablespoons maple syrup

1. To make the filling, place the pear slices in a large bowl. Add the sugar substitute, cornstarch, cinnamon, and nutmeg, and toss to coat the pears with the mixture.

2. Arrange a layer of pear slices in a spiral pattern over the bottom of the prepared crust. Continue building layers in this manner until all of the slices are used.

3. To make the syrup, place the cornstarch in a small saucepan. Slowly add the juice while stirring to dissolve the cornstarch. Stir in the maple syrup.

4. Place the saucepan over medium heat, and cook, stirring constantly, until the mixture begins to boil. Cook and stir for an additional minute, or until the mixture becomes clear and thickens. Drizzle the hot syrup over the top of the pie.

5. Cover the pie loosely with aluminum foil, and bake at 400°F for 15 minutes. Reduce the heat to 375°F, and bake for 40 additional minutes, or until the filling is bubbly. Remove the foil during the last 5 minutes of baking.

6. Allow the pie to cool for at least 1 hour before cutting into wedges and serving.

NUTRITIONAL FACTS (PER SLICE)

Calories: 197   Carbohydrate: 38 g   Cholesterol: 0 mg
Fat: 4.3 g   Fiber: 3.9 g   Protein: 2.6 g   Sodium: 75 mg

DIABETIC EXCHANGES: 1 Starch, 1$^1/_2$ Fruit, 1 Fat

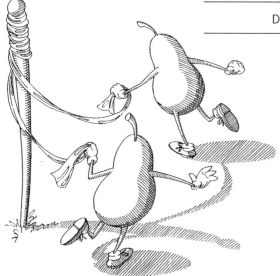

Raspberry Apple Turnovers

Yield: 12 turnovers

1. To make the filling, place the cornstarch and 1 tablespoon of the apple juice in a small bowl, and stir to mix well. Set aside.

2. Place the remaining 2 tablespoons of apple juice and the apples, raisins, and sugar in a small saucepan, and stir to mix. Cover and cook over medium-low heat for 5 to 7 minutes, stirring occasionally, until the apples are tender.

3. Stir the raspberries into the apple mixture, and cook uncovered for 1 or 2 minutes, or until the raspberries are soft and begin to break up. Stir in the cornstarch mixture, and cook for another minute or 2, stirring constantly, until the mixture is thickened and bubbly. Remove from the heat and set aside to cool to room temperature.

4. To make the pastry, place the flour, oat bran, sugar, and baking powder in a medium-sized bowl, and stir to mix well. Using a pastry cutter or 2 knives, cut in the margarine or butter until the mixture resembles coarse crumbs. Stir in just enough of the buttermilk to make a stiff dough that leaves the sides of the bowl and forms a ball.

5. Turn the dough onto a generously floured surface, and divide into 2 pieces. Using a rolling pin, roll each piece into an 8-x-12-inch rectangle. Using a knife or pizza wheel, cut each rectangle into six 4-inch squares.

6. Place a slightly rounded tablespoon of filling in the center of each square. Bring one corner over the filling and match up with the opposite corner to form a triangle. Seal the turnovers by crimping the edges with the tines of a fork. If necessary, dip the fork in sugar to prevent sticking.

7. To make the glaze, place the egg white and water in a small dish, and stir to mix.

8. Coat a large baking sheet with nonstick cooking spray. Using a spatula, transfer the pastries to the baking sheet. Brush the glaze mixture over the top of each pastry. Then sprinkle 1/4 teaspoon of sugar over the glaze.

9. Bake at 375°F for about 20 minutes, or until the edges are lightly browned. Transfer to a serving platter, and serve warm.

CRUSTS

1 1/4 cups unbleached flour

1 cup oat bran

2 tablespoons sugar

1/2 teaspoon baking powder

4 tablespoons chilled reduced-fat margarine or light butter, cut into pieces

1/2 cup plus 2 tablespoons nonfat or low-fat buttermilk

FILLING

1 tablespoon cornstarch

3 tablespoons apple juice, divided

1 1/4 cups finely chopped peeled fresh apples (about 2 medium)

1/4 cup golden raisins

2 tablespoons sugar

1/2 cup fresh or frozen (unthawed) raspberries

GLAZE

1 tablespoon beaten egg white

1 tablespoon water

1 tablespoon sugar

NUTRITIONAL FACTS (PER TURNOVER)

Calories: 132 Carbohydrate: 24 g Cholesterol: 0 mg
Fat: 2.7 g Fiber: 2.5 g Protein: 3.3 g Sodium: 74 mg

DIABETIC EXCHANGES: 1 Starch, 1/2 Fruit, 1/2 Fat

Mini Cherry Strudels

Yield: 24 pastries

CRUSTS

12 sheets (14 x 18 inches) phyllo pastry (about 10 ounces)

Butter-flavored cooking spray

FILLING

3 tablespoons sugar

2 tablespoons cornstarch

2 tablespoons white grape juice

1 bag (1 pound) frozen (unthawed) pitted cherries

Sugar substitute equal to 3 tablespoons sugar (page 19)

TOPPING

1½ teaspoons sugar

1½ teaspoons finely ground almonds

NUTRITIONAL FACTS (PER PASTRY)

Calories: 60 Carbohydrate: 12 g
Cholesterol: 0 mg   Fat: 1 g
Fiber: 0.5 g   Protein: 1 g
Sodium: 46 mg

DIABETIC EXCHANGES:
¾ Starch

---

1. To make the filling, place the sugar and cornstarch in a 1½-quart pot, and stir to mix well. Stir in first the juice, and then the cherries. Place the pot over medium heat, and cook, stirring constantly, for about 5 minutes, or until the cherries are thawed and the mixture is thickened and bubbly. Remove the pot from the heat, stir in the sugar substitute, and set aside to cool to room temperature.

2. To make the topping, place the sugar and almonds in a small bowl, and stir to mix well. Set aside.

3. Spread the phyllo dough out on a clean, dry surface, with the short end facing you. Cut the phyllo dough lengthwise down the center to make 2 stacks, each measuring about 18 x 7 inches. Lay one stack on top of the other to make one 18-x-7-inch stack of 24 phyllo sheets. Cover the dough with plastic wrap to prevent it from drying out as you work. (Remove strips as you need them, being sure to re-cover the remaining dough.)

4. Remove 1 strip of the phyllo dough, and lay it flat on a clean dry surface. Spray the strip lightly with cooking spray. Fold the bottom up to form a double layer of phyllo measuring approximately 9 x 7 inches.

5. Spread 1 level tablespoon of filling over the bottom of the phyllo sheet, leaving a 2-inch margin on each side. Fold the left and right edges inward to enclose the filling. Then roll the pastry up from the bottom, jelly-roll style. Repeat steps 4 and 5 with the remaining filling and phyllo sheets to make 24 strudels.

6. Coat a large baking sheet with nonstick cooking spray, and arrange the strudels on the sheets. Spray the top of each pastry lightly with cooking spray, and sprinkle each with ⅛ teaspoon of the almond mixture.

7. Bake at 375°F for about 15 minutes, or until lightly browned. Allow to cool for at least 15 minutes before serving. Serve warm or at room temperature.

Time-Saving Tip

To save time on the day you bake the pastries, prepare the strudels ahead of time to the point of baking, and arrange them in single layers in airtight containers, separating the layers with sheets of waxed paper. Then place the pastries in the freezer until needed. When ready to bake, arrange the frozen strudels on a coated sheet and allow them to sit at room temperature for 45 minutes before baking.

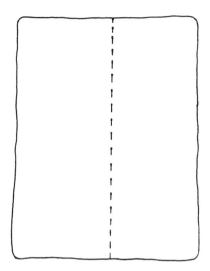

a. Cut the phyllo sheets into 2 long strips.

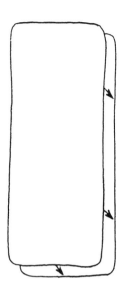

b. Lay 1 stack of strips on top of the other.

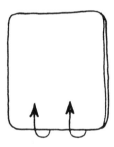

c. Fold the bottom of each strip up to double the strip.

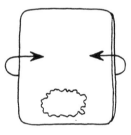

d. Spread the filling over the bottom of each strip. Fold the left and right edges inward.

Making Mini Cherry Strudels.

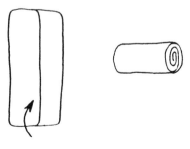

e. Roll the pastry up jelly-roll style.

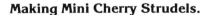

Flaky Apple Pastries

Yield: 40 pastries

CRUSTS

20 sheets (14 x 18 inches) phyllo pastry (about 1 pound)

$\frac{1}{2}$ cup plus 2 tablespoons reduced-fat margarine or light butter, melted

FILLING

5 cups finely chopped peeled apples (about 7 medium)

$\frac{1}{3}$ cup dark raisins or dried cranberries

1 cup apple juice, divided

2 tablespoons light brown sugar

1 teaspoon ground cinnamon

2 tablespoons cornstarch

TOPPING

1 tablespoon plus 2 teaspoons sugar

$\frac{1}{2}$ teaspoon ground cinnamon

1. To make the filling, place the apples, the raisins or dried cranberries, $\frac{3}{4}$ cup of the apple juice, the brown sugar, and the cinnamon in a 2-quart pot. Stir to mix well, and bring the mixture to a boil over high heat. Reduce the heat to low, cover, and simmer for about 5 minutes, or just until the apples lose their crispness.

2. In a small bowl, stir together the cornstarch and the remaining $\frac{1}{4}$ cup of apple juice. Add this mixture to the cooked apples, and stir over low heat for about 30 seconds, or until thickened. Set aside to cool to room temperature.

3. To make the topping, place the sugar and cinnamon in a small bowl, and stir to mix well. Set aside.

4. Spread the phyllo dough out on a clean, dry surface. Cut the dough lengthwise into 4 long strips, each measuring $3\frac{1}{2}$ x 18 inches. Cover the dough with plastic wrap to prevent it from drying out as you work. (Remove strips as you need them, being sure to re-cover the remaining dough.)

5. Remove 2 strips of phyllo dough and stack 1 on top of the other, laying the stack flat on a clean dry surface. Brush the top strip lightly with the melted margarine. Spread 1 level tablespoon of the filling over the bottom right-hand corner of the double phyllo strip. Fold the filled corner up and over to the left, so that the corner meets the left side of the strip. Continue folding in this manner until you form a triangle of dough. Repeat with the remaining filling and dough.

6. Coat a large baking sheet with nonstick cooking spray, and arrange the pastries seam side-down on the sheet. Brush the top of each pastry lightly with the melted margarine, and sprinkle each with $\frac{1}{8}$ teaspoon of the topping.

7. Bake at 375°F for 15 to 18 minutes, or until lightly browned. Allow to cool for at least 15 minutes before serving. Serve warm or at room temperature.

NUTRITIONAL FACTS (PER PASTRY)

Calories: 65   Carbohydrate: 11 g   Cholesterol: 0 mg
Fat: 1.5 g   Fiber: 0.5 g   Protein: 0.9 g   Sodium: 65 mg

DIABETIC EXCHANGES: $\frac{3}{4}$ Fruit, $\frac{1}{3}$ Fat

Time-Saving Tip

Like the Mini Cherry Strudels, these pastries can be prepared ahead of time to the point of baking, and then frozen until ready to bake. Just follow the directions on page 58.

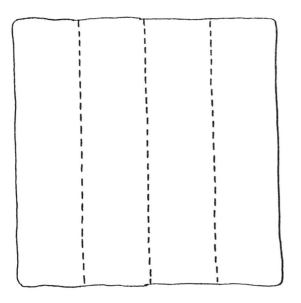 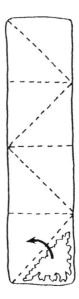

a. Cut the phyllo sheets into 4 strips.

b. Fold the filled corner up and over.

c. Continue folding to form a triangle.

Making Flaky Apple Pastries.

Greek Custard Pastries

Yield: 40 pastries

CRUSTS

20 sheets (14 X 18 inches) phyllo pastry (about 1 pound)

Butter-flavored cooking spray

¼ cup plus 1 tablespoon honey

FILLING

2 cups skim milk

⅓ cup quick-cooking Cream of Wheat cereal or farina

3 tablespoons sugar

¼ cup plus 2 tablespoons fat-free egg substitute

1 teaspoon vanilla extract

Sugar substitute equal to ¼ cup sugar (page 19)

1. To make the filling, place the milk in a 1½-quart pot. Cook over medium heat, stirring constantly, until the milk begins to boil. Whisk in the Cream of Wheat or farina and the sugar. Reduce the heat to low, and cook, still stirring, for 3 to 4 minutes, or until the mixture thickens slightly.

2. Slowly whisk the egg substitute into the cereal mixture. Continue to cook, still stirring, for an additional minute or 2, or until the mixture thickens slightly.

3. Remove the pot from the heat, and stir in the vanilla extract and sugar substitute. Transfer the mixture to a covered container, and refrigerate for at least 1 hour, or until the mixture is thoroughly chilled.

4. Spread the phyllo dough out on a clean, dry surface. Cut the dough lengthwise into 4 long strips, each measuring 3½ x 18 inches. Cover the dough with plastic wrap to prevent it from drying out as you work. (Remove strips as you need them, being sure to re-cover the remaining dough.)

5. Remove 1 strip of phyllo dough, and lay it flat on a clean dry surface. Spray the strip lightly with cooking spray. Lay another strip over the first, and spray lightly with cooking spray.

6. Spread 1 level tablespoon of the filling over the bottom right-hand corner of the double phyllo strip. Fold the filled corner up and over to the left, so that the corner meets the left side of the strip. Continue folding in this manner until you form a triangle of dough. Repeat with the remaining filling and dough. (See the figures on page 61 for clarification.)

7. Coat a large baking sheet with nonstick cooking spray. Arrange the pastries seam side-down on the sheet. Brush the top of each pastry with ¼ teaspoon of the honey.

8. Bake at 375°F for 15 minutes, or until lightly browned. Allow to cool for at least 15 minutes before serving. Serve warm.

NUTRITIONAL FACTS (PER PASTRY)
Calories: 54   Carbohydrate: 10 g   Cholesterol: 0 mg
Fat: 0.5 g   Fiber: 0.2 g   Protein: 1.4 g   Sodium: 56 mg

DIABETIC EXCHANGES: ⅔ Starch

4

Creamy Puddings, Mousses, and Trifles

Rich, creamy, and inviting, puddings are among the most popular of comfort foods. Puddings are versatile, too. Hearty noodle puddings and baked custards make healthful snacks, or can provide a sweet conclusion to a home-style family dinner. Elegant mousses and trifles fill the bill when you want a dessert for that special-occasion dinner. And, as you'll learn in other chapters, puddings also make deliciously smooth, creamy pie fillings.

Unfortunately, most puddings and mousses are loaded with an unhealthy amount of fat and sugar. In traditional recipes, whole milk, cream, egg yolks, and sugar top the list of ingredients. Consider, for instance, a traditionally prepared dish of chocolate mousse. Believe it or not, just one serving can contain up to eight teaspoons of sugar and twenty-five grams of fat!

The good news is that puddings are among the easiest of foods to prepare with little or no sugar or fat. This chapter offers a pleasing assortment of creamy desserts, ranging from an elegant Mocha Mousse to a homey Cherry Cheese Kugel.

These treats are suited for a variety of occasions, and can easily be worked into your meal plans by using milk, starch, and fruit exchanges.

How have sugar and fat been reduced without sacrificing creamy consistency and great taste? As you will see, these recipes often combine small amounts of sugar with noncaloric sweeteners so that you get optimal sweetness, flavor, and texture with a lot less sugar than that in traditional recipes. Often, fresh fruit and fruit juices add further sweetness. In fact, most of these recipes contain less than 3 teaspoons of sugar per serving. Fat is kept to an absolute minimum by using skim milk, nonfat yogurt, nonfat ricotta cheese, nonfat cream cheese, and other nonfat dairy products. The result is a selection of low-sugar, low-fat desserts that are as high in nutrition as they are tempting and flavorful.

But the proof is in the pudding. So whip up a creamy dish of comfort, and enjoy a treat that is so satisfyingly sweet, even you will find it hard to believe that it's also guilt-free!

Getting the Fat Out of Your Pudding Recipes

It's a shame that most pudding recipes are so high in fat and cholesterol, as, when properly prepared, pudding makes a great low-fat snack or dessert. Happily, it's easy to do a healthful makeover of any pudding. Use this table to replace high-fat ingredients like cream and eggs with low-fat and no-fat ingredients. You'll find that any pudding can be made ultra-light without sacrificing the creamy richness you love.

Substitutions That Save Fat

Instead of:	Use:	You Save:	Special Considerations:
1 cup whole milk.	1 cup skim milk.	65 calories, 8 g fat, 30 mg cholesterol.	For extra richness, add 2 tablespoons of instant nonfat dry milk powder to each cup of skim milk.
	1 cup 1% low-fat milk.	50 calories, 6 g fat, 25 mg cholesterol.	For extra richness, add 2 tablespoons of instant nonfat dry milk powder to each cup of low-fat milk.
1 cup cream.	$\frac{2}{3}$ cup nonfat ricotta cheese blended with $\frac{1}{3}$ cup skim milk until smooth.	674 calories, 88 g fat, 300 mg cholesterol.	Use this ingredient only in uncooked puddings and mousses.
	1 cup evaporated skimmed milk.	622 calories, 88 g fat, 330 mg cholesterol.	This ingredient may be used in cooked puddings and custards.
	1 cup skim milk mixed with $\frac{1}{3}$ cup instant nonfat dry milk powder.	622 calories, 88 g fat, 330 mg cholesterol.	This ingredient may be used in cooked puddings and custards.
1 cup regular cream cheese.	1 cup nonfat cream cheese.	600 calories, 80 g fat, 200 mg cholesterol.	For best results, use a firm block-style nonfat cream cheese.
	1 cup reduced-fat (Neufchâtel) cream cheese.	240 calories, 26 g fat, 48 mg cholesterol.	
1 cup sour cream	1 cup nonfat sour cream.	252 calories, 48 g fat, 70 mg cholesterol.	Some brands of sour cream will separate when heated. Choose a brand like Land O Lakes, which is heat-stable, if the sour cream will be used in a cooked pudding.

Instead of:	Use:	You Save:	Special Considerations:
1 cup sour cream.	1 cup plain nonfat yogurt.	355 calories, 48 g fat, 75 mg cholesterol.	All yogurts will separate if heated. To prevent this, stir 2 tablespoons of flour or 1 tablespoon of cornstarch into each cup of yogurt before adding it to the cooked pudding.
1 cup whipped cream or regular whipped topping.	1 cup light whipped topping.	136 calories, 16 g fat, 160 mg cholesterol.	Evaporated skimmed milk or a fat-free mixture that contains gelatin may also be whipped to add volume to mousses, reducing the need for whipped cream. (See the inset on page 77 for details.)
1 cup butter or margarine.	$\frac{1}{2}$ cup Butter Buds liquid.	1,500 calories, 176 g fat, 528 mg cholesterol.*	Butter Buds may be used as an ingredient in a pudding base.
	$\frac{3}{4}$ cup reduced-fat margarine or light butter.	800–1,200 calories, 88–112 g fat, 264–528 mg cholesterol.*	Nonfat margarines generally do not melt well enough to be used in cooking and baking.
1 large egg.	3 tablespoons fat-free egg substitute.	60 calories, 5 g fat, 210 mg cholesterol.	
1 egg yolk.	1 tablespoon fat-free egg substitute.	40 calories, 5 g fat, 210 mg cholesterol.	
1 ounce baking chocolate.	3 tablespoons cocoa powder plus 1 tablespoon water or another liquid.	111 calories, 13.5 g fat.	

*The cholesterol comparison applies to butter only, as all margarines are cholesterol-free.

Creamy Tapioca Pudding

Yield: 5 servings

1. Place the milk and nonfat dry milk powder in a 2-quart pot, and stir to dissolve the milk powder. Stir in the tapioca.

2. Stirring constantly, bring the mixture to a boil over medium heat. Reduce the heat to low and simmer for 5 minutes, stirring occasionally, until the tapioca becomes translucent. Stir in the sugar.

3. Place the egg substitute in a small bowl, and stir in $\frac{1}{2}$ cup of the hot tapioca mixture. Return the mixture to the pot, and cook over low heat, stirring constantly, for 2 additional minutes, or until the mixture thickens slightly. Do not let the mixture boil.

4. Remove the pot from the heat, and stir in the vanilla extract and sugar substitute. Allow the pudding to cool for 15 minutes.

5. Divide the warm pudding among five 8-ounce serving dishes, and chill for several hours, or until thick and creamy. (The mixture will thicken as it cools.) Top each serving with a pinch of nutmeg, and serve immediately, refrigerating any leftovers.

3 cups skim milk

$\frac{1}{2}$ cup instant nonfat dry milk powder

$\frac{1}{3}$ cup small pearl tapioca

$\frac{1}{4}$ cup sugar

$\frac{1}{2}$ cup fat-free egg substitute

1 teaspoon vanilla extract

Sugar substitute equal to 2 tablespoons sugar (page 19)

Ground nutmeg (garnish)

NUTRITIONAL FACTS (PER $\frac{3}{4}$-CUP SERVING)

Calories: 163 Carbohydrate: 30 g Cholesterol: 4 mg
Fat: 0.3 g Fiber: 0.1 g Protein: 10 g Sodium: 153 mg

DIABETIC EXCHANGES: 1 Starch, 1 Skim Milk

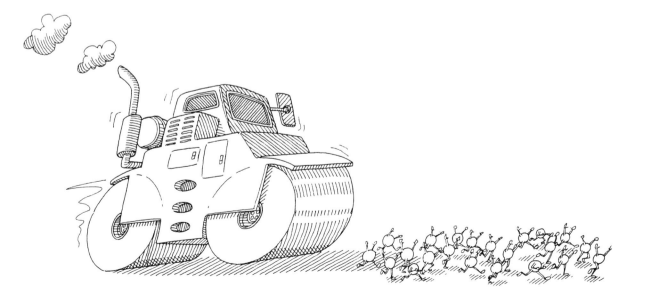

Pineapple Tapioca Pudding

Yield: 6 servings

2½ cups skim milk

⅓ cup instant nonfat dry milk powder

¼ cup plus 2 tablespoons small pearl tapioca

¼ cup sugar

½ cup plus 2 tablespoons fat-free egg substitute

1 can (8 ounces) crushed pineapple in juice, undrained

1 teaspoon vanilla extract

Sugar substitute equal to 2 tablespoons sugar (page 19)

1. Place the milk and nonfat dry milk powder in a 2-quart pot, and stir to dissolve the milk powder. Stir in the tapioca.

2. Stirring constantly, bring the mixture to a boil over medium heat. Reduce the heat to low and simmer for 5 minutes, stirring occasionally, until the tapioca becomes translucent. Stir in the sugar.

3. Place the egg substitute in a small bowl, and stir in ½ cup of the hot tapioca mixture. Return the mixture to the pot, and cook over low heat, stirring constantly, for 2 additional minutes, or until the mixture thickens slightly. Do not let the mixture boil.

4. Remove the pot from the heat, and stir in the pineapple, including the juice, and the vanilla extract and sugar substitute. Allow the pudding to cool for 15 minutes.

5. Divide the warm pudding among six 8-ounce serving dishes, and chill for several hours, or until thick and creamy. (The mixture will thicken as it cools.) Serve chilled, refrigerating any leftovers.

NUTRITIONAL FACTS (PER ¾-CUP SERVING)

Calories: 151 Carbohydrate: 30 g Cholesterol: 2 mg
Fat: 0.2 g Fiber: 0.3 g Protein: 7.5 g Sodium: 115 mg

DIABETIC EXCHANGES: ½ Starch, 1 Fruit, ½ Skim Milk

Rice Pudding With Raspberry Sauce

Yield: 8 servings

½ cup uncooked short grain white rice

½ cup pear nectar

1¼ cups water, divided

¼ cup plus 2 tablespoons sugar

2 envelopes unflavored gelatin

1 cup skim milk

1 cup nonfat sour cream

1½ teaspoons vanilla extract

1 cup light whipped topping

1. Place the rice, nectar, and ¾ cup of the water in a 1½-quart pot, and bring to a boil over high heat. Reduce the heat to low, stir once, and cover. Simmer for 20 minutes, or until the rice is tender and most of the liquid has been absorbed. Remove the pot from the heat, uncover, and allow to cool to room temperature.

2. Combine the sugar and the remaining ½ cup of water in a 1-quart pot. Sprinkle the gelatin over the top, and set aside for 2 minutes to allow the gelatin to soften. Place the pot over low heat, and cook, stirring constantly, for 3 minutes, or until the gelatin and sugar are completely dissolved. Remove the pot from the heat, and stir in the milk.

3. Transfer the gelatin mixture to a large bowl, and chill for about 25 minutes, or until the mixture has the consistency of raw egg whites. Using an electric mixer, beat the chilled gelatin mixture at high speed for about 4 minutes, or until it resembles soft whipped cream.

4. Place the cooled rice mixture, sour cream, and vanilla extract in a medium-sized bowl, and stir to mix well. Fold the rice mixture into the whipped gelatin mixture. Gently fold in the whipped topping.

5. Divide the pudding among eight 10-ounce balloon wine glasses. Chill the desserts for at least 2 hours, or until firm.

6. While the pudding is chilling, make the sauce by placing the cornstarch in a 1-quart saucepan. Stir in first the nectar, and then the raspberries. Bring the mixture to a boil over medium heat, stirring constantly. Continue to cook and stir for about 2 minutes, or until the raspberries break up. Remove the pot from the heat, and stir in the sugar substitute. Transfer to a covered container, and chill for at least 1 hour.

7. When ready to serve, spoon 2 tablespoons of the chilled sauce over the top of each pudding. Serve immediately, refrigerating any leftovers.

SAUCE

2 teaspoons cornstarch

$\frac{1}{3}$ cup pear nectar

2 cups fresh or frozen (unthawed) raspberries

Sugar substitute equal to $\frac{1}{4}$ cup sugar (page 19)

NUTRITIONAL FACTS (PER $\frac{7}{8}$-CUP SERVING)

Calories: 176   Carbohydrate: 36 g   Cholesterol: 1 mg
Fat: 1.3 g   Fiber: 1.5 g   Protein: 4.7 g   Sodium: 66 mg

DIABETIC EXCHANGES: 1 Starch, 1 Fruit, $\frac{1}{3}$ Skim Milk

---

Apple-Raisin Bread Pudding

1. Cut the bread into $\frac{1}{2}$-inch cubes, and measure the cubes. There should be 6 cups. (Adjust the amount if necessary.)

2. Place the bread cubes in a large bowl. Add the apples and raisins, and toss to mix. Set aside.

3. Place the sugar and cinnamon in a medium-sized bowl, and stir to mix well. Add the milk, egg substitute, and vanilla extract, and stir to mix well. Pour the milk mixture over the bread cube mixture, and stir gently to mix. Let the mixture sit at room temperature for 10 minutes.

4. Coat a 1$\frac{1}{2}$-quart casserole dish with nonstick cooking spray, and pour the bread mixture into the dish. Place the dish in a pan filled with 1 inch of hot water.

Yield: 8 servings

6 slices stale multigrain or whole wheat bread

1$\frac{1}{4}$ cups chopped peeled apple

$\frac{1}{4}$ cup dark raisins

$\frac{1}{4}$ cup plus 2 tablespoons sugar

$\frac{1}{2}$ teaspoon ground cinnamon

2 cups skim milk

$\frac{3}{4}$ cup fat-free egg substitute

1$\frac{1}{2}$ teaspoons vanilla extract

5. Bake uncovered at 350°F for 1 hour and 10 minutes, or until a sharp knife inserted in the center of the dish comes out clean. Allow the pudding to cool at room temperature for at least 20 minutes. Serve warm or at room temperature, refrigerating any leftovers.

NUTRITIONAL FACTS (PER ¾-CUP SERVING)

Calories: 189   Carbohydrate: 37 g   Cholesterol: 1 mg
Fat: 0.8 g   Fiber: 2.5 g   Protein: 8 g   Sodium: 198 mg

DIABETIC EXCHANGES: 1 Starch, 1 Fruit, ½ Skim Milk

Old-Fashioned Rice Pudding

Yield: 12 servings

½ cup plus 2 tablespoons uncooked short grain white rice

¾ cup pear or apricot nectar

½ cup water

1 quart skim milk

½ cup sugar

½ cup instant nonfat dry milk powder

1 cup fat-free egg substitute

2 teaspoons vanilla extract

½ cup dried cherries, dried cranberries, or dark raisins

¼ teaspoon ground nutmeg

1. Place the rice, nectar, and water in a 4-quart pot, and bring to a boil over high heat. Reduce the heat to low, stir once, and cover. Simmer for 15 minutes, or until the rice is almost tender and most of the liquid has been absorbed.

2. Add the milk, sugar, and nonfat dry milk to the rice mixture, and cook over medium heat, stirring constantly, until the mixture just begins to boil. Reduce the heat to low.

3. Place the egg substitute in a small bowl, and stir in ½ cup of the hot rice mixture. Return the mixture to the pot, and continue cooking and stirring for 2 to 3 minutes, or until the pudding thickens slightly. (Do not let the mixture boil.) Remove the pot from the heat, and stir in the vanilla extract and dried fruit.

4. Coat a 2½-quart round casserole dish with nonstick cooking spray. Pour the pudding into the dish, and sprinkle with the nutmeg. Place the dish in a pan filled with 1 inch of hot water.

5. Bake uncovered at 350°F for 1 hour and 10 minutes, or until a sharp knife inserted midway between the rim of the dish and the center comes out clean. Allow the pudding to cool at room temperature for 45 minutes. Serve warm, or refrigerate for several hours and serve chilled. Refrigerate any leftovers.

NUTRITIONAL FACTS (PER ⅔-CUP SERVING)

Calories: 148   Carbohydrate: 29 g   Cholesterol: 2 mg
Fat: 0.3 g   Fiber: 0.5 g   Protein: 7 g   Sodium: 95 mg

DIABETIC EXCHANGES: 1 Starch, ½ Fruit, ½ Skim Milk

Creamy Baked Custard

1. Place all of the ingredients except for the nutmeg in a blender or food processor, and blend for 30 seconds to mix well.

2. Coat a 1½-quart casserole dish with nonstick cooking spray. Pour the custard mixture into the dish, and sprinkle with the nutmeg. Place the dish in a pan filled with 1 inch of hot water.

3. Bake uncovered at 350°F for about 1 hour and 20 minutes, or until set. When done, a sharp knife inserted midway between the center of the custard and the rim of the dish should come out clean. Allow the custard to cool at room temperature for 30 minutes. Then cover and chill for several hours or overnight before serving. Refrigerate any leftovers.

Yield: 6 servings

2 cups skim milk

1 cup evaporated skimmed milk

1 cup fat-free egg substitute

½ cup sugar

2 teaspoons vanilla extract

Ground nutmeg

NUTRITIONAL FACTS (PER ⅔-CUP SERVING)

Calories: 146 Carbohydrate: 26 g Cholesterol: 3 mg
Fat: 0.2 g Fiber: 0 g Protein: 10 g Sodium: 158 mg

DIABETIC EXCHANGES: 1 Starch, ¾ Skim Milk

Baked Pumpkin Custard

1. Place all of the ingredients in a blender or food processor, and process until smooth.

2. Coat a 2-quart soufflé dish with nonstick cooking spray, and pour the custard mixture into the dish. Place the dish in a pan filled with 1 inch of hot water.

3. Bake uncovered at 350°F for about 1 hour and 15 minutes, or until a sharp knife inserted in the center of the custard comes out clean. Allow the custard to cool at room temperature for 30 minutes. Then cover and chill for at least 8 hours or overnight before serving. Refrigerate any leftovers.

Yield: 8 servings

1½ cups mashed cooked or canned pumpkin

1 can (12 ounces) evaporated skimmed milk

1¾ cups fat-free egg substitute

⅓ cup orange juice

½ cup light brown sugar

1½ teaspoons vanilla extract

1½ teaspoons pumpkin pie spice

NUTRITIONAL FACTS (PER ⅔-CUP SERVING)

Calories: 131 Carbohydrate: 23 g Cholesterol: 1 mg
Fat: 0.2 g Fiber: 1.3 g Protein: 9 g Sodium: 131 mg

DIABETIC EXCHANGES: 1 Starch, ½ Skim Milk

Polenta Pudding

Yield: 8 servings

¼ cup plus 2 tablespoons whole grain cornmeal

2½ cups skim milk

1 cup evaporated skimmed milk

¼ cup plus 2 tablespoons honey

1 cup fat-free egg substitute

1½ teaspoons vanilla extract

⅓ cup golden raisins

Ground nutmeg (garnish)

1. Place the cornmeal in a 2½-quart pot, and slowly stir in the milk and the evaporated milk. Cook over medium heat, stirring constantly, for 10 to 12 minutes, or until the mixture comes to a boil. Reduce the heat to low, and continue cooking and stirring for 2 additional minutes, or until slightly thickened. Slowly stir in the honey.

2. Place the egg substitute in a small bowl, and stir in 1 cup of the hot cornmeal mixture. Slowly stir the egg mixture into the pudding, and continue cooking and stirring for 2 minutes, or until slightly thickened. Remove the pot from the heat, and stir in the vanilla extract and raisins.

3. Coat a 1½-quart round casserole dish with nonstick cooking spray. Pour the pudding mixture into the dish, and sprinkle with the nutmeg. Place the dish in a pan filled with 1 inch of hot water.

4. Bake uncovered at 350°F for 1 hour, or until set. When done, a sharp knife inserted midway between the center of the pudding and the rim of the dish should come out clean. Allow the pudding to cool at room temperature for at least 30 minutes. Serve warm, or refrigerate for several hours and serve chilled. Refrigerate any leftovers.

NUTRITIONAL FACTS (PER ⅔-CUP SERVING)

Calories: 156   Carbohydrate: 30 g   Cholesterol: 2 mg
Fat: 0.5 g   Fiber: 0.8 g   Protein: 9 g   Sodium: 150 mg

DIABETIC EXCHANGES: 1 Starch, ½ Fruit, ½ Skim Milk

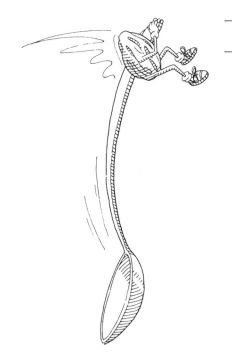

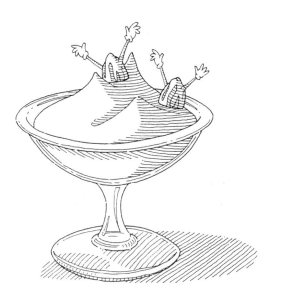

Cherry Cheese Kugel

Yield: 8 servings

1. Cook the noodles until tender according to package directions. Drain, rinse with cool water, and drain again. Set aside.

2. Place the cream cheese and sugar in a large bowl, and stir to mix well. Add the cottage cheese, egg substitute, and vanilla extract, and stir to mix well. Gently stir in first the noodles, and then the cherries. Set aside.

3. To make the topping, place the sugar and almonds in a small bowl, and stir to mix well.

4. Coat a 1½-quart casserole dish with nonstick cooking spray, and spread the noodle mixture evenly in the dish. Sprinkle the topping over the noodle mixture.

5. Bake at 350°F for 1 hour, or until bubbly around the edges and lightly browned on top. Allow the kugel to cool at room temperature for at least 30 minutes before serving. Serve warm or at room temperature, refrigerating any leftovers.

4 ounces medium or wide no-yolk egg noodles

1 block (8 ounces) nonfat cream cheese, softened to room temperature

¼ cup plus 2 tablespoons sugar

1 cup dry curd or nonfat cottage cheese

1 cup fat-free egg substitute

1½ teaspoons vanilla extract

1½ cups fresh or frozen (thawed) pitted sweet cherries, halved

TOPPING

1 tablespoon sugar

2 tablespoons finely ground almonds

NUTRITIONAL FACTS (PER ⅔-CUP SERVING)

Calories: 179 Carbohydrate: 27 g Cholesterol: 3 mg
Fat: 1.4 g Fiber: 1.2 g Protein: 13 g Sodium: 188 mg

DIABETIC EXCHANGES: ½ Starch, ½ Fruit, 1 Skim Milk

Spiced Pumpkin Mousse

Yield: 4 servings

1. Place the pudding mix, pumpkin, milk, and pumpkin pie spice in a medium-sized bowl, and stir to mix well. Using a wire whisk or electric mixer, beat the mixture for 2 minutes, or until well mixed. Place the mixture in the refrigerator for 10 minutes, or until thickened.

2. Gently fold the whipped topping into the pumpkin mixture. Divide the mixture among four 8-ounce wine glasses, and chill for at least 1 hour before serving. Serve chilled, refrigerating any leftovers.

1 package (4-serving size) instant sugar-free butterscotch pudding mix

1¼ cups mashed cooked or canned pumpkin

1¼ cups skim milk

1½ teaspoons pumpkin pie spice

1½ cups light whipped topping

NUTRITIONAL FACTS (PER 1-CUP SERVING)

Calories: 121 Carbohydrate: 22 g Cholesterol: 1 mg
Fat: 2.8 g Fiber: 2.1 g Protein: 4 g Sodium: 207 mg

DIABETIC EXCHANGES: 1 Starch, ½ Skim Milk, ½ Fat

Mocha Mousse

Yield: 6 servings

1 cup skim milk, divided

1 envelope unflavored gelatin

1/2 cup instant nonfat dry milk powder

1/4 cup sugar

1 1/2 cups nonfat ricotta cheese

1/4 cup coffee liqueur

1/4 cup cocoa powder

Sugar substitute equal to 1/4 cup sugar (page 19)

1 teaspoon vanilla extract

1 cup light whipped topping

TOPPING

1/4 cup plus 2 tablespoons light whipped topping

1/2 teaspoon cocoa powder

1. Place 1/2 cup of the milk in a 1-quart pot. Sprinkle the gelatin over the milk, and set aside for 2 minutes to allow the gelatin to soften.

2. Place the gelatin mixture over low heat, and cook, stirring constantly, for about 3 minutes, or until the gelatin is completely dissolved. (Do not let the mixture boil.) Remove the pot from the heat, and stir in the remaining 1/2 cup of milk, the nonfat dry milk, and the sugar.

3. Transfer the gelatin mixture to a medium-sized mixing bowl, and chill for about 25 minutes, or until the mixture has the consistency of raw egg whites. Using an electric mixer, beat the chilled gelatin mixture at high speed for about 4 minutes, or until it resembles soft whipped cream.

4. While the gelatin mixture is chilling, place the ricotta, liqueur, cocoa, sugar substitute, and vanilla extract in a food processor or blender, and process until smooth. Gently fold the ricotta mixture into the whipped gelatin mixture. Then fold in the whipped topping.

5. Divide the mousse among six 10-ounce balloon wine glasses. Chill for at least 2 hours, or until firm. When ready to serve, top each mousse with a tablespoon of light whipped topping and a sprinkling of cocoa powder. Serve immediately, refrigerating any leftovers.

NUTRITIONAL FACTS (PER 1-CUP SERVING)

Calories: 194 Carbohydrate: 28 g Cholesterol: 12 mg
Fat: 2.5 g Fiber: 1.2 g Protein: 14 g Sodium: 150 mg

DIABETIC EXCHANGES: 1 Starch, 1 Skim Milk, 1/2 Fat

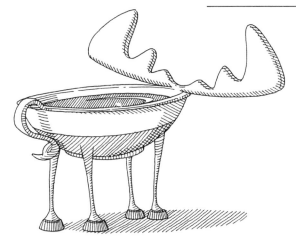

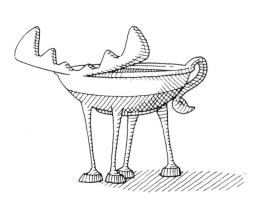

Strawberry-Cheese Mousse

Yield: 8 servings

1. Place the gelatin and sugar in a large heatproof bowl, and stir to mix well. Pour the boiling water over the gelatin mixture, and stir until the gelatin and sugar are completely dissolved. Set aside to cool to room temperature.

2. While the gelatin mixture is cooling, place the cream cheese, ricotta, sugar substitute, and $\frac{1}{2}$ cup of the mashed strawberries in a food processor or blender, and process until smooth. Set aside.

3. Using an electric mixer, beat the cooled gelatin mixture for about 3 minutes, or until it has the consistency of soft whipped cream. Gently fold the cheese mixture into the gelatin mixture. Then fold in first the remaining cup of mashed strawberries, and then the whipped topping.

4. Divide mixture among eight 10-ounce balloon wine glasses. Chill for at least 2 hours, or until firm. When ready to serve, top each mousse with one whole strawberry. Serve immediately, refrigerating any leftovers.

1 package (4-serving size) sugar-free strawberry gelatin mix

$\frac{1}{3}$ cup sugar

$\frac{3}{4}$ cup boiling water

1 block (8 ounces) nonfat cream cheese

1 cup nonfat ricotta cheese

Sugar substitute equal to $\frac{1}{4}$ cup sugar (page 19)

$1\frac{1}{2}$ cups mashed fresh strawberries (about 3 cups sliced), divided

$1\frac{1}{4}$ cups light whipped topping

TOPPING

8 large whole fresh strawberries

NUTRITIONAL FACTS (PER 1-CUP SERVING)

Calories: 127   Carbohydrate: 19 g   Cholesterol: 7 mg
Fat: 1.5 g   Fiber: 1.1 g   Protein: 10 g   Sodium: 186 mg

DIABETIC EXCHANGES: $\frac{1}{2}$ Fruit, 1 Skim Milk

Banana Pudding Parfaits

Yield: 4 servings

1. Use the skim milk to prepare the pudding according to package directions. Cover the mixture and chill for at least 30 minutes, or until set.

2. To assemble the parfaits, place 2 tablespoons of the pudding in the bottom of each of four 8-ounce wine or parfait glasses. Top with 2 tablespoons of banana slices. Then crumble $1\frac{1}{2}$ vanilla wafers over the bananas. Finally, layer 3 tablespoons of pudding over the wafers. Repeat the banana, vanilla wafer, and pudding layers, and serve immediately, refrigerating any leftovers.

2 cups skim or 1-percent low-fat milk

1 package (4-serving size) instant sugar-free vanilla pudding

1 cup sliced bananas (about 1 large)

12 reduced-fat vanilla wafers

NUTRITIONAL FACTS (PER SERVING)

Calories: 151   Carbohydrate: 30 g   Cholesterol: 2 mg
Fat: 1.7 g   Fiber: 1 g   Protein: 5.3 g   Sodium: 260 mg

DIABETIC EXCHANGES: 1 Starch, $\frac{1}{2}$ Fruit, $\frac{1}{2}$ Skim Milk

Razzleberry Trifle

Yield: 10 servings

2½ cups sliced fresh strawberries

1 cup fresh or frozen (thawed) raspberries

Sugar substitute equal to 2 tablespoons sugar (page 19)

3 cups skim milk

1 package (6-serving size) instant or cook-and-serve sugar-free vanilla pudding mix

10 slices (½-inch each) fat-free loaf cake

¼ cup low-sugar raspberry jam

TOPPING

1 cup light whipped topping

¾ cup sugar-free nonfat vanilla yogurt

1. Place the strawberries, raspberries, and sugar substitute in a medium-sized bowl, and stir to mix well. Set the mixture aside for 20 minutes to let the juices develop.

2. Use the skim milk to prepare the pudding according to package directions. Set aside. (If you are using cook-and-serve pudding, chill the pudding for at least 2 hours before proceeding with the recipe.)

3. Spread one side of each cake slice with a thin layer of the jam. Arrange half of the cake slices, jam side up, over the bottom of a 3-quart trifle bowl or another decorative glass bowl. Top first with half of the fruit, and then with half of the pudding. Repeat the cake, fruit, and pudding layers.

4. To make the topping, place the whipped topping in a small bowl, and fold the yogurt into the topping. Swirl the mixture over the top of the trifle. Cover and chill for at least 2 hours before serving. Refrigerate any leftovers.

NUTRITIONAL FACTS (PER 1-CUP SERVING)

Calories: 161 Carbohydrate: 33 g Cholesterol: 2 mg
Fat: 1.2 g Fiber: 1.2 g Protein: 5.6 g Sodium: 222 mg

DIABETIC EXCHANGES: 1 Starch, 1 Fruit, ⅓ Skim Milk

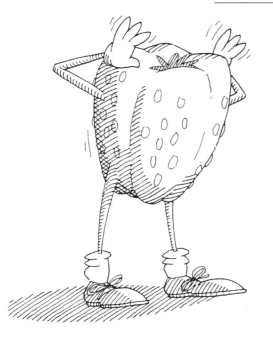

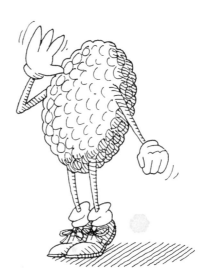

Chocolate Raspberry Trifle

Yield: 12 servings

1. Use the skim milk to prepare the pudding according to package directions. Cover the pudding, and refrigerate for at least 2 hours, or until well chilled, before assembling the trifle.

2. Place the berries and sugar substitute in a small bowl, and mash with a fork. Set aside.

3. Cut the angel food cake into $1\frac{1}{2}$-inch cubes, and place the cubes in a large bowl. Add the chilled pudding, and toss gently to coat the cake with the pudding.

4. Arrange half of the cake mixture evenly in the bottom of a 3-quart trifle bowl or another decorative glass bowl. Top with half of the fruit. Repeat the cake and fruit layers.

5. To make the topping, place the whipped topping in a small bowl, and fold the yogurt into the topping. Swirl the mixture over the top of the trifle. Cover and chill for at least 2 hours before serving. Refrigerate any leftovers.

3 cups skim milk

1 package (6-serving size) instant or cook-and-serve sugar-free dark or white chocolate pudding mix

2 cups fresh or frozen (thawed) raspberries

Sugar substitute equal to 2 tablespoons sugar (page 19)

1 large angel food cake ($1\frac{1}{4}$ pounds)

TOPPING

2 cups light whipped topping

$\frac{1}{2}$ cup sugar-free nonfat vanilla yogurt

NUTRITIONAL FACTS (PER SERVING)

Calories: 205 Carbohydrate: 39 g Cholesterol: 1 mg
Fat: 2.8 g Fiber: 1.5 g Protein: 6 g Sodium: 352 mg

DIABETIC EXCHANGES: 1 Starch, 1 Fruit, $\frac{1}{2}$ Skim Milk, $\frac{1}{2}$ Fat

---

FAT-FIGHTING TIP

Creamy Lightness With Less Whipped Cream

Creamy, light-as-air mousses, puddings, and pie fillings often get their lightness—and much of their fat—from whipped cream. But you can have a light and creamy texture, with far less fat, if you whip the gelatin, as is done in the Mocha Mousse (page 74) and Strawberry-Cheese Mousse (page 75) recipes. Whipping gelatin incorporates air into the mixture, making it light and fluffy. This reduces the need for ingredients like fatty whipped cream. For delightfully airy mousses and pie fillings, whip the gelatin mixture for 2 to 4 minutes, or until it has the consistency of soft whipped cream. Then, to eliminate even more fat, replace the whipped cream with one-half to two-thirds as much light whipped topping.

Phyllo Custard Cups

Yield: 6 servings

CRUSTS

4 sheets (14 x 18 inches) phyllo
    pastry (about 3¼ ounces)

Butter-flavored cooking spray

4 teaspoons sugar

FILLING

2¼ cups skim milk

¼ cup plus 1 tablespoon
    quick-cooking Cream of Wheat
    cereal or farina

½ cup plus 1 tablespoon fat-free
    egg substitute

Sugar substitute equal to ¼ cup
    sugar (page 19)

3 tablespoons finely chopped
    dried apricots

⅛ teaspoon ground nutmeg

½ teaspoon almond extract

SYRUP

3 tablespoons orange juice

¾ teaspoon cornstarch

3 tablespoons honey

1. To make the crusts, spread the phyllo dough out on a clean dry surface. Cover the dough with plastic wrap to prevent it from drying out as you work. (Remove sheets as you need them, being sure to re-cover the remaining dough.)

2. Remove 1 sheet of phyllo dough, and lay it on a clean dry surface. Spray the sheet lightly with the cooking spray, and sprinkle with 1 teaspoon of the sugar. Top with another phyllo sheet, spray with cooking spray, and sprinkle with another teaspoon of sugar. Repeat with the 2 remaining sheets.

3. Cut the stack of phyllo sheets lengthwise into two 18-inch-long strips. Then cut each strip crosswise to make 3 pieces, each measuring approximately 6 x 7 inches. You should now have 6 stacks of phyllo squares, each 4 layers thick.

4. Coat six jumbo muffin cups or six 6-ounce custard cups with nonstick cooking spray. Gently press 1 stack of phyllo squares into each cup, pleating as necessary to make it fit. Press the corners back slightly.

5. Bake at 350°F for about 8 minutes, or until golden brown. Remove the crusts from the oven and let sit for 5 minutes. Transfer the crusts to wire racks to cool completely. (Note that the crusts may be prepared the day before you plan to serve the dessert, and stored in an airtight container until ready to use.)

6. To make the filling, place the milk in a 1½-quart pot. Place the pot over medium heat, and cook, stirring constantly, until the milk begins to boil. Whisk in the cereal, reduce the heat to low, and cook, still stirring, for 3 to 4 additional minutes, or until the mixture thickens slightly.

7. Place the egg substitute in a small bowl, and stir in ½ cup of the hot milk mixture. Return the mixture to the pot, and cook, stirring constantly, for 2 minutes, or until the mixture thickens slightly. Do not let the mixture boil.

8. Remove the pot from the heat, and stir in the sugar substitute, apricots, nutmeg, and almond extract. Allow the custard to cool at room temperature for 15 minutes.

9. To make the syrup, place the orange juice and cornstarch in a small saucepan, and stir to mix well. Stir in the honey. Place over medium-low heat, and cook, stirring constantly, until the mixture begins to boil. Continue to cook, still stirring, for another minute, or until the mixture thickens slightly. Remove the pot from the heat and set aside.

10. To assemble the desserts, stir the custard, and place $\frac{1}{2}$ cup of the warm mixture in each crust. Drizzle 1 tablespoon of the hot syrup over the custard and the edges of the pastry. Serve immediately. (Leftovers should be refrigerated, but may become soggy.)

NUTRITIONAL FACTS (PER SERVING)

Calories: 154   Carbohydrate: 27 g   Cholesterol: 1 mg
Fat: 1.4 g   Fiber: 0.6 g   Protein: 6 g   Sodium: 142 mg

DIABETIC EXCHANGES: 1 Starch, $\frac{1}{2}$ Fruit, $\frac{1}{2}$ Skim Milk

---

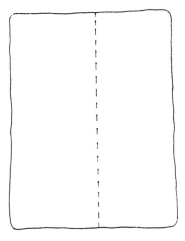

a. Cut the phyllo sheets into 2 long strips.

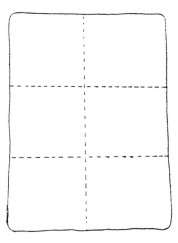

b. Cut each strip crosswise to make 3 squares.

Making Phyllo Custard Cups.

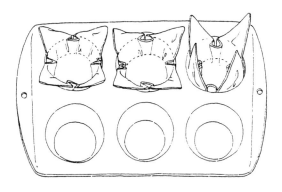

c. Press 1 stack of squares into each muffin cup.

Tiramisu Treats

Yield: 4 servings

4 slices (¾-inch each) fat-free loaf cake

BERRY MIXTURE

1½ cups fresh or frozen (thawed) strawberries

Sugar substitute equal to 1 tablespoon sugar (page 19)

RICOTTA MIXTURE

1¼ cups nonfat ricotta cheese

Sugar substitute equal to 2 tablespoons plus 2 teaspoons sugar (page 19)

¾ teaspoon vanilla extract

LIQUEUR MIXTURE

2 tablespoons plus 2 teaspoons coffee liqueur

1 teaspoon cocoa powder

TOPPING

¼ cup plus 2 tablespoons light whipped topping

¼ teaspoon cocoa powder

1. To make the berry mixture, place the berries and sugar substitute in a small bowl, and mash with a fork. Set aside.

2. To make the ricotta mixture, place the ricotta, sugar substitute, and vanilla extract in a food processor, and process until smooth. Set aside.

3. To make the liqueur mixture, combine the liqueur and cocoa in a small bowl, and stir to mix well. Set aside.

4. To assemble the desserts, crumble a half slice of the cake into the bottom of each of four 10-ounce balloon wine glasses. Top the cake with 1½ tablespoons of the berry mixture, 2½ tablespoons of the ricotta mixture, and 1 teaspoon of the liqueur mixture. Repeat the layers, and top each dessert with 1½ tablespoons of the whipped topping and a sprinkling of cocoa. Serve immediately, refrigerating any leftovers.

NUTRITIONAL FACTS (PER SERVING)

Calories: 159   Carbohydrate: 23 g   Cholesterol: 12 mg
Fat: 1.1 g   Fiber: 1.2 g   Protein: 12.3 g   Sodium: 302 mg

DIABETIC EXCHANGES: ½ Starch, ½ Fruit, 1 Skim Milk

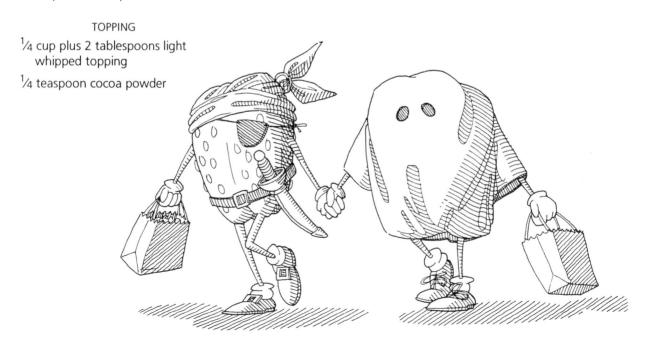

5

Colossal Cookies

Cookies are the perfect treat when you crave a bite of something sweet. A crisp, crunchy biscotti is just the right accompaniment to a steaming cup of coffee. And a soft oatmeal cookie makes a satisfyingly chewy mid-morning snack.

Unfortunately, most cookies tend to contain higher proportions of fat and sugar than other sweet treats do, and so have no place in a diabetic diet—or in any other diet, for that matter. Does this mean that you must give up these toothsome treats, or compromise on quality? Absolutely not! When made properly, cookies can provide both good nutrition and great taste with a minimum of fat and sugar. The proof is in the recipes presented in this chapter. Unlike most cookie recipes, these feature wholesome ingredients like whole wheat flour, oat bran, and wheat germ. Just as important, these recipes keep fat to a minimum. Healthful additions like fruit juice concentrates, puréed fruits, and sweet potatoes replace much of the fat, and at the same time reduce the need for refined sugar. Two other handy ingredients—reduced-fat margarine and light butter—also slash the fat, while helping these confections retain the texture that you love.

What about sugar? It is almost impossible to make a good cookie without at least some sugar, as sugar adds not just sweetness, but also texture. In the past, many diabetic recipes eliminated most of the sugar, and used artificial sweeteners instead. However, to obtain the desired consistency, these recipes usually had to include an unhealthy amount of fat.

In accordance with the new diabetic dietary guidelines, the recipes in this chapter do contain sugar, although they provide at least 25 percent less than most traditional recipes do. The inclusion of fruits; of spices like vanilla and nutmeg; and of mildly sweet grains like oats and oat bran, reduce the need for added sugar while keeping the cookies sweet and flavorful.

The nutrition analysis provided for each recipe will allow you to easily fit these treats into your meal plan. For instance, most of these cookies count for one or even just a half of a starch exchange each. This means that you can save one of your starch exchanges from dinner, and then enjoy a temptingly sweet, guilt-free treat that would satisfy even the most discriminating of cookie monsters.

Colossal Chocolate Chippers

1. Place the margarine or butter and the brown sugar in the bowl of a food processor or electric mixer, and process until smooth. Add the egg substitute and vanilla extract, and process until smooth.

2. Place the flour, baking soda, and baking powder in a medium-sized bowl, and stir to mix well. Add the flour mixture to the margarine mixture, and process to mix well. Stir in the chocolate chips and walnuts.

3. Coat a baking sheet with nonstick cooking spray. Drop rounded teaspoonfuls of the dough onto the sheet, spacing them 1½ inches apart.

4. Bake at 300°F for 16 to 18 minutes, or until golden brown. Cool the cookies on the pan for 1 minute. Then transfer the cookies to wire racks, and cool completely. Serve immediately, or transfer to an airtight container.

Yield: 42 cookies

¼ cup plus 2 tablespoons reduced-fat margarine or light butter

¾ cup plus 2 tablespoons light brown sugar

3 tablespoons fat-free egg substitute

1 teaspoon vanilla extract

1¼ cups whole wheat pastry flour

½ teaspoon baking soda

½ teaspoon baking powder

½ cup chocolate chips

½ cup chopped walnuts

NUTRITIONAL FACTS (PER COOKIE)

Calories: 50   Carbohydrate: 7 g   Cholesterol: 0 mg
Fat: 2.3 g   Fiber: 0.6 g   Protein: 1.1 g   Sodium: 30 mg

DIABETIC EXCHANGES (PER COOKIE): ½ Starch, ½ Fat

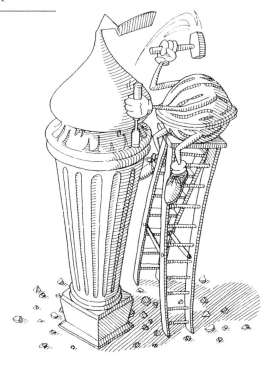

Chocolate-Chocolate Chippers

Yield: 42 cookies

¼ cup plus 2 tablespoons reduced-fat margarine or light butter

¾ cup plus 2 tablespoons light brown sugar

3 tablespoons fat-free egg substitute

1 teaspoon vanilla extract

1 cup whole wheat pastry flour

¼ cup Dutch processed cocoa powder

½ teaspoon baking soda

½ teaspoon baking powder

½ cup chocolate chips

½ cup chopped pecans, walnuts, or almonds

1. Place the margarine or butter and the brown sugar in the bowl of a food processor or electric mixer, and process until smooth. Add the egg substitute and vanilla extract, and process until smooth.

2. Place the flour, cocoa, baking soda, and baking powder in a medium-sized bowl, and stir to mix well. Add the flour mixture to the margarine mixture, and process to mix well. Stir in the chocolate chips and nuts.

3. Coat a baking sheet with nonstick cooking spray. Drop rounded teaspoonfuls of the dough onto the sheet, spacing them 1½ inches apart.

4. Bake at 300°F for 16 to 18 minutes, or until golden brown. Cool the cookies on the pan for 1 minute. Then transfer the cookies to wire racks, and cool completely. Serve immediately, or transfer to an airtight container.

NUTRITIONAL FACTS (PER COOKIE)

Calories: 49 Carbohydrate: 7 g Cholesterol: 0 mg
Fat: 2.4 g Fiber: 0.7 g Protein: 1 g Sodium: 30 mg

DIABETIC EXCHANGES: ½ Starch, ½ Fat

Golden Oatmeal Cookies

1. Place the margarine or butter and the brown sugar in the bowl of a food processor or electric mixer, and process until smooth. Add the egg substitute and vanilla extract, and process until smooth.

2. Place the flour, oats, baking soda, and baking powder in a medium-sized bowl, and stir to mix well. Add the flour mixture to the margarine mixture, and process to mix well. Stir in the raisins or other fruit and the nuts.

3. Coat a baking sheet with nonstick cooking spray. Drop rounded teaspoonfuls of dough onto the sheet, spacing them $1\frac{1}{2}$ inches apart. Flatten each cookie slightly with the tip of a spoon.

4. Bake at 300°F for 16 to 18 minutes, or until golden brown. Cool the cookies on the pan for 1 minute. Then transfer the cookies to wire racks, and cool completely. Serve immediately, or transfer to an airtight container.

Yield: 45 cookies

$\frac{1}{2}$ cup reduced-fat margarine or light butter

1 cup light brown sugar

3 tablespoons fat-free egg substitute

1 teaspoon vanilla extract

1 cup whole wheat pastry flour

1 cup quick-cooking oats

$\frac{3}{4}$ teaspoon baking soda

$\frac{1}{2}$ teaspoon baking powder

$\frac{1}{2}$ cup dark raisins, dried cranberries, or chopped dried fruit

$\frac{1}{2}$ cup chopped walnuts, pecans, or almonds

NUTRITIONAL FACTS (PER COOKIE)

Calories: 52   Carbohydrate: 8 g   Cholesterol: 0 mg
Fat: 2 g   Fiber: 0.7 g   Protein: 1.1 g   Sodium: 37 mg

DIABETIC EXCHANGES: $\frac{1}{2}$ Starch, $\frac{1}{3}$ Fat

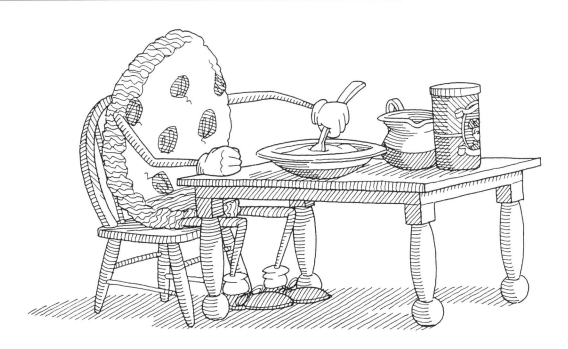

Cinnamon-Raisin Drops

Yield: 42 cookies

¼ cup plus 2 tablespoons reduced-fat margarine or light butter

¾ cup plus 2 tablespoons light brown sugar

3 tablespoons fat-free egg substitute

1 teaspoon vanilla extract

1¼ cups whole wheat pastry flour

½ teaspoon baking soda

½ teaspoon baking powder

1¼ teaspoons ground cinnamon

½ cup dark raisins

½ cup chopped walnuts

1. Place the margarine or butter and the brown sugar in the bowl of a food processor or electric mixer, and process until smooth. Add the egg substitute and vanilla extract, and process until smooth.

2. Place the flour, baking soda, baking powder, and cinnamon in a medium-sized bowl, and stir to mix well. Add the flour mixture to the margarine mixture, and process to mix well. Stir in the raisins and walnuts.

3. Coat a baking sheet with nonstick cooking spray. Drop rounded teaspoonfuls of the dough onto the sheet, spacing them 1½ inches apart.

4. Bake at 300°F for 16 to 18 minutes, or until golden brown. Cool the cookies on the pan for 1 minute. Then transfer the cookies to wire racks, and cool completely. Serve immediately, or transfer to an airtight container.

NUTRITIONAL FACTS (PER COOKIE)
Calories: 46   Carbohydrate: 7 g   Cholesterol: 0 mg
Fat: 1.8 g   Fiber: 0.6 g   Protein: 1 g   Sodium: 30 mg

DIABETIC EXCHANGES: ½ Starch, ⅓ Fat

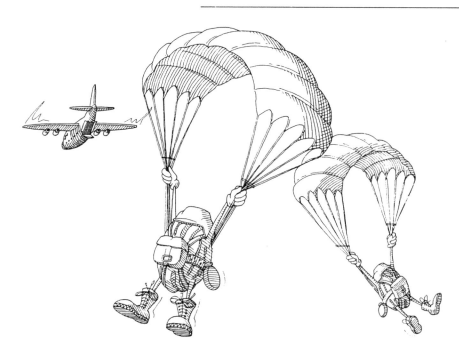

Cranberry-Orange Cookies

Yield: 38 cookies

1. Place the margarine or butter and the sugar in the bowl of a food processor or electric mixer, and process until smooth. Add the egg white, juice concentrate, and vanilla extract, and process until smooth.

2. Place the flour, oat bran, baking soda, and orange rind in a medium-sized bowl, and stir to mix well. Add the flour mixture to the margarine mixture, and process to mix well. Add the cranberries and pecans, and process just enough to mix in.

3. Coat a baking sheet with nonstick cooking spray. Using your hands, shape the dough into 1-inch balls and arrange the balls on the sheet, spacing them 1½ inches apart. (If the dough is too sticky to handle, place it in the freezer for a few minutes.) Using the bottom of a glass dipped in sugar, flatten the cookies to ¼-inch thickness.

4. Bake at 275°F for 22 to 25 minutes. To check for doneness, lift a cookie from the sheet with a spatula. The bottom should be golden brown. Cool the cookies on the pan for 1 minute. Then transfer the cookies to wire racks, and cool completely. Serve immediately, or transfer to an airtight container and arrange in single layers separated by sheets of waxed paper.

¼ cup margarine or butter

½ cup plus 2 tablespoons sugar

1 egg white

2 tablespoons plus 2 teaspoons frozen orange juice concentrate, thawed

1 teaspoon vanilla extract

1½ cups unbleached flour

½ cup oat bran

1 teaspoon baking soda

1 teaspoon dried grated orange rind

¾ cup fresh or frozen (unthawed) cranberries, coarsely chopped

½ cup chopped toasted pecans (see inset below)

NUTRITIONAL FACTS (PER COOKIE)

Calories: 58 Carbohydrate: 8.5 g Cholesterol: 0 mg
Fat: 2.4 g Fiber: 0.5 g Protein: 1 g Sodium: 45 mg

DIABETIC EXCHANGES: ½ Starch, ½ Fat

Getting the Most Out of Nuts

Nuts add crunch, great taste, and essential nutrients to all kinds of baked goods. Unfortunately, they also add fat. But you can halve the fat—without halving the taste—simply by toasting nuts before adding them to your recipe. Toasting intensifies the flavor of nuts so much that you can often cut the amount used in half. Simply arrange the nuts in a single layer on a baking sheet, and bake at 350°F for about 10 minutes, or until lightly browned with a toasted, nutty smell. To save time, toast a large batch and store leftovers in an airtight container in the refrigerator for several weeks, or keep them in the freezer for several months.

Sweet Potato-Pecan Cookies

Yield: 40 cookies

1 1/2 cups whole wheat pastry flour

3/4 cup oat bran

1/2 cup plus 2 tablespoons dark brown sugar

3/4 teaspoon baking soda

1 teaspoon dried grated orange rind

1/2 cup plus 2 tablespoons mashed cooked or canned sweet potato

1/4 cup plus 1 tablespoon frozen orange juice concentrate, thawed

40 small pecan halves

1. Place the flour, oat bran, brown sugar, baking soda, and orange rind in a medium-sized bowl, and stir to mix well.

2. Place the sweet potato and juice concentrate in a small bowl, and stir to mix well. Add the sweet potato mixture to the flour mixture, and stir to mix well. (Note that the mixture will seem dry at first, but will form a stiff dough as you keep stirring.)

3. Coat a baking sheet with nonstick cooking spray. Using your hands, roll the dough into 1-inch balls and arrange the balls on the sheet, spacing them 1 1/2 inches apart. (If the dough is too sticky to handle, place it in the freezer for a few minutes.) Press a pecan half into the center of each cookie to flatten.

4. Bake at 275°F for about 18 minutes, or until lightly browned. Cool the cookies on the pan for 1 minute. Then transfer the cookies to wire racks, and cool completely. Serve immediately, or transfer to an airtight container and arrange in single layers separated by sheets of waxed paper.

NUTRITIONAL FACTS (PER COOKIE)

Calories: 47 Carbohydrate: 7.5 g Cholesterol: 0 mg
Fat: 1.5 g Fiber: 1 g Protein: 1.2 g Sodium: 27 mg

DIABETIC EXCHANGES: 1/2 Starch, 1/3 Fat

Old-Fashioned Peanut Butter Cookies

Yield: 42 cookies

1/2 cup plus 2 tablespoons creamy peanut butter

3/4 cup light brown sugar

1/2 cup unsweetened applesauce or apricot baby food

2 teaspoons vanilla extract

1 3/4 cups whole wheat pastry flour

3/4 teaspoon baking soda

1. Place the peanut butter and brown sugar in the bowl of a food processor or electric mixer, and process until smooth. Add the applesauce or apricots and the vanilla extract, and process until smooth.

2. Place the flour and baking soda in a medium-sized bowl, and stir to mix well. Add the flour mixture to the peanut butter mixture, and process until the dough is well mixed and forms a ball.

3. Coat a baking sheet with nonstick cooking spray. Using your hands, shape the dough into 1-inch balls, and arrange the balls on the baking sheet, spacing them 1 1/2 inches apart. (If the dough is too sticky to handle, place it in the freezer for a few minutes.) Press the tines of a fork in a crisscross pattern on the top of each ball, flattening it to 1/4-inch thickness. (Dip the fork in sugar between cookies to prevent sticking.)

4. Bake at 325°F for 10 to 12 minutes. To check for doneness, lift a cookie from the sheet with a spatula. The bottom should be golden brown. Cool the cookies on the pan for 1 minute. Then transfer the cookies to wire racks, and cool completely. Serve immediately, or transfer to an airtight container.

NUTRITIONAL FACTS (PER COOKIE)

Calories: 49 Carbohydrate: 7.1 g Cholesterol: 0 mg
Fat: 1.9 g Fiber: 0.7 g Protein: 1.4 g Sodium: 32 mg

DIABETIC EXCHANGES: $\frac{1}{2}$ Starch, $\frac{1}{3}$ Fat

Mocha-Almond Cookies

Yield: 45 cookies

1. Place the margarine or butter and the brown sugar in the bowl of a food processor or electric mixer, and process until smooth. Add the egg white and extracts, and process until smooth.

2. Place the flour, oat bran, cocoa, coffee granules, and baking soda in a medium-sized bowl, and stir to mix well. Add the flour mixture to the margarine mixture, and process until well mixed.

3. Using your hands, shape the dough into 1-inch balls. (If the dough is too sticky to handle, place it in the freezer for a few minutes.) Place the nuts in a small flat dish, and roll the balls in the nuts to coat all sides.

4. Coat a baking sheet with nonstick cooking spray, and arrange the balls on the prepared sheet, spacing them $1\frac{1}{2}$ inches apart. Using the bottom of a glass, flatten each ball to $\frac{1}{4}$-inch thickness.

5. Bake at 300°F for 16 to 18 minutes. To check for doneness, lift a cookie from the sheet with a spatula. The bottom should be golden brown. Cool the cookies on the pan for 1 minute. Then transfer the cookies to wire racks, and cool completely. Serve immediately, or transfer to an airtight container.

$\frac{1}{2}$ cup reduced-fat margarine or light butter

1 cup light brown sugar

1 egg white

1 teaspoon vanilla extract

1 teaspoon almond extract

$1\frac{1}{2}$ cups whole wheat pastry flour

$\frac{2}{3}$ cup oat bran

$\frac{1}{4}$ cup plus 2 tablespoons cocoa powder

$1\frac{1}{2}$ teaspoons instant coffee granules

$\frac{3}{4}$ teaspoon baking soda

$\frac{2}{3}$ cup finely ground almonds

NUTRITIONAL FACTS (PER COOKIE)

Calories: 50 Carbohydrate: 8 g Cholesterol: 0 mg
Fat: 2 g Fiber: 1.1 g Protein: 1.4 g Sodium: 33 mg

DIABETIC EXCHANGES: $\frac{1}{2}$ Starch, $\frac{1}{3}$ Fat

Brown Sugar and Spice Cookies

Yield: 42 cookies

¼ cup margarine or butter

1 cup light brown sugar

¼ cup apricot baby food or
   mashed bananas

1 egg white

2 teaspoons vanilla extract

1 cup oat bran

1½ cups whole wheat pastry flour

1 teaspoon baking soda

¾ teaspoon ground cinnamon

½ teaspoon ground allspice

42 pecan halves (optional)*

*By adding the pecans, you'll add
10 calories and 1 gram of fat per
cookie.

1. Place the margarine or butter and the brown sugar in the bowl of a food processor or electric mixer, and process until smooth. Add the apricots or bananas, egg white, and vanilla extract, and process until smooth.

2. Place the oat bran, flour, baking soda, and spices in a medium-sized bowl, and stir to mix well. Add the oat bran mixture to the margarine mixture, and process until the dough is well mixed and forms a ball. (Add a little more apricot or banana if the mixture seems too dry.)

3. Coat a baking sheet with nonstick cooking spray. Using your hands, shape the dough into 1-inch balls and arrange the balls on the sheet, spacing them 1½ inches apart. (If the dough is too sticky to handle, place it in the freezer for a few minutes.) Using the bottom of a glass dipped in sugar, flatten each ball to ¼-inch thickness. Alternatively, press a pecan half into the center of each cookie to flatten.

4. Bake at 300°F for 16 to 18 minutes. To check for doneness, lift a cookie from the sheet with a spatula. The bottom should be golden brown. Cool the cookies on the pan for 1 minute. Then transfer the cookies to wire racks, and cool completely. Serve immediately, or transfer to an airtight container.

NUTRITIONAL FACTS (PER COOKIE)

Calories: 43   Carbohydrate: 8 g   Cholesterol: 0 mg
Fat: 1.3 g   Fiber: 0.9 g   Protein: 1 g   Sodium: 42 mg

DIABETIC EXCHANGES: ½ Starch, ¼ Fat

Orange-Molasses Cookies

1. Place the margarine or butter and the sugar in the bowl of a food processor or electric mixer, and process until smooth. Add the molasses, egg white, and orange juice, and process until smooth.

2. Place the flour, oat bran, baking soda, and orange rind in a medium-sized bowl, and stir to mix well. Add the flour mixture to the margarine mixture, and process until the dough is well mixed and forms a ball. (If the dough seems too dry, add a little more orange juice.)

3. Coat a baking sheet with nonstick cooking spray. Using your hands, roll the dough into 1-inch balls and arrange the balls on the sheet, spacing them 1½ inches apart. (If the dough is too sticky to handle, place it in the freezer for a few minutes.) Using the bottom of a glass dipped in sugar, flatten each ball to ¼-inch thickness.

4. Bake at 300°F for about 14 minutes. To check for doneness, lift a cookie from the sheet with a spatula. The bottom should be lightly browned. Cool the cookies on the pan for 1 minute. Then transfer the cookies to wire racks, and cool completely. Serve immediately, or transfer to an airtight container.

Yield: 40 cookies

¼ cup margarine or butter

¾ cup plus 2 tablespoons light brown sugar

¼ cup molasses

1 egg white

2 tablespoons orange juice

1½ cups whole wheat pastry flour

⅔ cup oat bran

¾ teaspoon baking soda

1½ teaspoons dried grated orange rind

NUTRITIONAL FACTS (PER COOKIE)
Calories: 42   Carbohydrate: 7.5 g   Cholesterol: 0 mg
Fat: 1.2 g   Fiber: 0.8 g   Protein: 1 g   Sodium: 36 mg

DIABETIC EXCHANGES: ½ Starch, ¼ Fat

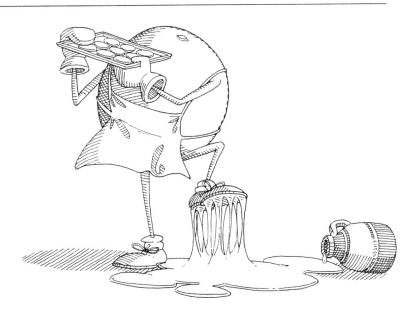

Whole Wheat Ginger Snaps

Yield: 45 cookies

¼ cup margarine or butter

1 cup light brown sugar

¼ cup unsweetened applesauce

1 egg white

2 teaspoons vanilla extract

2⅓ cups whole wheat pastry flour

1 teaspoon baking soda

2 teaspoons ground ginger

1 teaspoon ground cinnamon

1.   Place the margarine or butter and the brown sugar in the bowl of a food processor or electric mixer, and process until smooth. Add the applesauce, egg white, and vanilla extract, and process until smooth.

2.   Place the flour, baking soda, and spices in a medium-sized bowl, and stir to mix well. Add the flour mixture to the margarine mixture, and process until the dough is well mixed and forms a ball. (Add a little more applesauce if the dough seems too dry.)

3.   Coat a baking sheet with nonstick cooking spray. Using your hands, shape the dough into 1-inch balls and arrange the balls on the sheet, spacing them 1½ inches apart. (If the dough is too sticky to handle, place it in the freezer for a few minutes.) Using the bottom of a glass dipped in sugar, flatten each ball to ¼-inch thickness.

4.   Bake at 300°F for about 15 minutes. To check for doneness, lift a cookie from the sheet with a spatula. The bottom should be lightly browned. Cool the cookies on the pan for 1 minute. Then transfer the cookies to wire racks, and cool completely. Serve immediately, or transfer to an airtight container.

NUTRITIONAL FACTS (PER COOKIE)
Calories: 43   Carbohydrate: 8 g   Cholesterol: 0 mg
Fat: 1.1 g   Fiber: 0.8 g   Protein: 0.9 g   Sodium: 39 mg

DIABETIC EXCHANGES: ½ Starch, ¼ Fat

Pecan Puffs

Yield: 24 cookies

2 large egg whites, warmed to room temperature

⅛ teaspoon cream of tartar

⅛ teaspoon salt

¼ cup plus 2 tablespoons sugar

½ teaspoon vanilla extract

½ cup pecan halves

For best results, make these light-as-air treats on a dry day. Also, be careful to prevent any egg yolk from getting mixed in with the whites, or the whites will not whip properly.

1.   Place the egg whites in the bowl of an electric mixer, and beat on high until foamy. Add the cream of tartar and salt, and continue beating until soft peaks form. Still beating, slowly add first the sugar, 1 tablespoon at a time, and then the vanilla extract. Beat the mixture just until stiff peaks form when the beaters are raised. Remove the beaters, and fold in the pecan halves.

2. Line a large baking sheet with aluminum foil. (Do not grease the sheet or coat it with cooking spray.) Drop heaping teaspoonfuls of the mixture onto the baking sheet, spacing them 1½ inches apart.

3. Bake at 250°F for about 45 minutes, or until firm and creamy white. Turn the oven off, and let the puffs cool in the oven for 2 hours with the door closed. Remove the pans from the oven, and peel the puffs from the foil. Serve immediately, or transfer to an airtight container.

NUTRITIONAL FACTS (PER COOKIE)

Calories: 29 Carbohydrate: 3.5 g Cholesterol: 0 mg
Fat: 1.4 g Fiber: 0.2 g Protein: 0.5 g Sodium: 15 mg

DIABETIC EXCHANGES: ¼ Starch, ¼ Fat

Mint Chocolate Meringues

Like the Pecan Puffs (above), these delicate cookies should be baked on a dry day.

Yield: 24 cookies

2 large egg whites, warmed to room temperature

¼ teaspoon cream of tartar

⅛ teaspoon salt

¼ cup plus 2 tablespoons sugar

2 tablespoons cocoa powder

¾ teaspoon vanilla extract

½ cup mint chocolate chips

1. Place the egg whites in the bowl of an electric mixer, and beat on high until foamy. Add the cream of tartar and salt, and continue beating until soft peaks form. Still beating, slowly add the sugar, 1 tablespoon at a time. Then beat in first the cocoa, 1 tablespoon at a time, and then the vanilla extract. Beat the mixture just until stiff peaks form when the beaters are raised. Remove the beaters, and fold in the chocolate chips.

2. Line a large baking sheet with aluminum foil. (Do not grease the sheet or coat it with cooking spray.) Drop heaping teaspoonfuls of the mixture onto the baking sheet, spacing them 1 inch apart.

3. Bake at 250°F for about 45 minutes, or until firm. Turn the oven off, and let the meringues cool in the oven for 2 hours with the door closed. Remove the pans from the oven, and peel the meringues from the foil. Serve immediately, or transfer to an airtight container.

NUTRITIONAL FACTS (PER COOKIE)

Calories: 31 Carbohydrate: 5 g Cholesterol: 0 mg
Fat: 1.1 g Fiber: 0.3 g Protein: 0.5 g Sodium: 15 mg

DIABETIC EXCHANGES: ⅓ Starch, ¼ Fat

Dutch Chocolate Pinwheels

Yield: 64 cookies

½ cup reduced-fat margarine or
   light butter

1½ cups sugar

3 tablespoons fat-free egg
   substitute

2 teaspoons vanilla extract

1½ cups unbleached flour

1½ cups oat flour

¾ teaspoon baking soda

¼ cup Dutch processed cocoa
   powder

1 tablespoon plus 2 teaspoons
   chocolate syrup

1. Place the margarine or butter and the sugar in the bowl of a food processor or electric mixer, and process until smooth. Add the egg substitute and vanilla extract, and process until smooth.

2. Place the flours and baking soda in a medium-sized bowl, and stir to mix well. Add the flour mixture to the margarine mixture, and process until the dough is well mixed and forms a ball that leaves the sides of the bowl. (If the dough seems too dry, add a little more egg substitute. If it seems too sticky, add a little more unbleached flour.)

3. Remove half of the dough, and set aside. Add the cocoa and chocolate syrup to the remaining dough, and process to mix well.

4. Coat two 12-inch square pieces of waxed paper with nonstick cooking spray. Divide the white dough into 2 pieces. Lay 1 piece of the white dough on top of 1 of the sheets of waxed paper, and pat it into a 4-x-6-inch rectangle. Top with the other sheet of waxed paper, and, using a rolling pin, roll the dough into a 6-x-8-inch rectangle. Next, divide the chocolate dough into 2 pieces and, in the same manner, roll 1 piece of the chocolate dough into a 6-x-8-inch rectangle.

5. Peel the waxed paper off the rectangles of dough, and lay the chocolate rectangle on top of the white rectangle. Roll the double layer of dough up from the long end, jelly-roll style. Wrap the roll in waxed paper and freeze for at least 3 hours, or until ready to bake. Repeat this procedure with the remaining pieces of dough.

6. When ready to bake, coat a baking sheet with nonstick cooking spray. Slice the frozen dough into ¼-inch-thick pieces, and arrange the slices on the sheet, spacing them 1½ inches apart.

7. Bake at 300°F for 12 to 14 minutes. To check for doneness, lift a cookie from the sheet with a spatula. The bottom should be lightly browned. Cool the cookies on the pan for 1 minute. Then transfer the cookies to wire racks, and cool completely. Serve immediately, or transfer to an airtight container.

NUTRITIONAL FACTS (PER COOKIE)

Calories: 46   Carbohydrate: 9 g   Cholesterol: 0 mg
Fat: 0.8 g   Fiber: 0.5 g   Protein: 0.8 g   Sodium: 23 mg

DIABETIC EXCHANGES: ⅔ Starch

Hamantaschen

Yield: 40 cookies

1. To make the filling, place the dried fruit, water, and honey in a small saucepan, and stir to mix. Bring to a boil over high heat. Reduce the heat to low, cover, and simmer, stirring occasionally, for about 20 minutes, or until the liquid has been absorbed. Remove the pan from the heat, and allow the filling to cool to room temperature.

2. To make the glaze, place the egg white and water in a small bowl, and stir to mix well. Set aside.

3. To make the pastry, place the margarine or butter and the sugar in the bowl of an electric mixer, and beat until smooth. Add the egg whites, and beat until smooth.

4. Place the flours and baking powder in a medium-sized bowl, and stir to mix well. Add the flour mixture to the margarine mixture, and beat until the dough leaves the sides of the bowl and forms a ball. Cover the bowl with plastic wrap to prevent it from drying out.

5. Place a fourth of the dough on a floured surface, and roll into a 10-inch circle of $\frac{1}{16}$-inch thickness. (Chill the dough for a few minutes if it is too sticky to handle.) Using the rim of a 3-inch glass or a 3-inch round cookie cutter, cut out 10 rounds of dough.

6. Brush a small amount of glaze around the outer edges of each circle. Place 1 teaspoon of filling in the center of each round, and fold up 3 sides of each circle about $\frac{1}{2}$ inch to form a tricorn—a 3-sided hat. Repeat with the remaining dough and filling to make 40 pastries.

7. Coat a baking sheet with nonstick cooking spray, and transfer the pastries to the sheet. Brush some glaze over each pastry, and bake at 325°F for about 20 minutes, or until golden brown. Transfer the pastries to wire racks, and cool completely. Serve immediately, or transfer to an airtight container.

PASTRY

$\frac{1}{4}$ cup plus 1 tablespoon reduced-fat margarine or light butter

$\frac{1}{4}$ cup plus 2 tablespoons sugar

3 egg whites

1 $\frac{1}{4}$ cups whole wheat pastry flour

1 $\frac{1}{4}$ cups unbleached flour

1 $\frac{1}{2}$ teaspoons baking powder

FILLING

1 cup finely chopped dried apricots, prunes, or other dried fruit

1 cup water

2 tablespoons honey

GLAZE

2 tablespoons beaten egg white

1 teaspoon water

NUTRITIONAL FACTS (PER COOKIE)

Calories: 53   Carbohydrate: 10 g   Cholesterol: 0 mg
Fat: 0.8 g   Fiber: 0.8 g   Protein: 1.4 g   Sodium: 35 mg

DIABETIC EXCHANGES: $\frac{1}{3}$ Starch, $\frac{1}{3}$ Fruit

Chocolate-Pecan Biscotti

Yield: 24 biscotti

¾ cup plus 2 tablespoons
  unbleached flour

¾ cup whole wheat pastry flour

⅔ cup sugar

¼ cup plus 2 tablespoons Dutch
  processed cocoa powder

2 teaspoons baking powder

¼ cup reduced-fat margarine or
  light butter, cut into pieces

¼ cup toasted chopped pecans
  (page 87)

¼ cup plus 2 tablespoons fat-free
  egg substitute

2 teaspoons vanilla extract

1. Place the flours, sugar, cocoa, and baking powder in a large bowl, and stir to mix well. Using a pastry cutter or 2 knives, cut in the margarine or butter until the mixture resembles coarse meal. Stir in the nuts. Add the egg substitute and vanilla extract, and stir just until the mixture holds together.

2. Turn the dough onto a lightly floured surface, divide it in half, and shape each half into a 9-x-2-inch log. Coat a baking sheet with nonstick cooking spray, and place the logs on the sheet, leaving 4 inches of space between them to allow for spreading. Bake at 350°F for about 25 minutes, or until lightly browned.

3. Cool the logs at room temperature for 10 minutes. Place the logs on a cutting board, and use a serrated knife to slice them diagonally into ½-inch-thick slices.

4. Reduce the oven temperature to 300°F. Return the slices to the baking sheet, arranging them in a single layer, cut side down. Bake for 10 minutes. Then turn the slices over, and bake for 10 additional minutes, or until dry and crisp.

5. Transfer the biscotti to wire racks, and cool completely. Serve immediately, or store in an airtight container.

NUTRITIONAL FACTS (PER BISCOTTI)

Calories: 72   Carbohydrate: 13 g   Cholesterol: 0 mg
Fat: 2 g   Fiber: 1 g   Protein: 1.7 g   Sodium: 45 mg

DIABETIC EXCHANGES: 1 Starch, ⅓ Fat

Poppy Seed-Almond Biscotti

1. Place the flours, sugar, and baking powder in a large bowl, and stir to mix well. Using a pastry cutter or 2 knives, cut in the margarine or butter until the mixture resembles coarse meal. Stir in the almonds and poppy seeds. Add the egg substitute and extracts, and stir just until the mixture holds together.

2. Turn the dough onto a lightly floured surface, divide it in half, and shape each half into a 9-x-2-inch log. Coat a baking sheet with nonstick cooking spray, and place the logs on the sheet, leaving 4 inches of space between them to allow for spreading. Bake at 350°F for about 25 minutes, or until lightly browned.

3. Cool the logs at room temperature for 10 minutes. Place the logs on a cutting board, and use a serrated knife to slice the logs diagonally into $\frac{1}{2}$-inch-thick slices.

4. Reduce the oven temperature to 300°F. Return the slices to the baking sheet, arranging them in a single layer, cut side down. Bake for 10 minutes. Then turn the slices over, and bake for 10 additional minutes, or until dry and crisp.

5. Transfer the biscotti to wire racks, and cool completely. Serve immediately, or store in an airtight container.

1 cup unbleached flour

1 cup whole wheat pastry flour

$\frac{2}{3}$ cup sugar

2 teaspoons baking powder

$\frac{1}{4}$ cup reduced-fat margarine or light butter, cut into pieces

$\frac{1}{4}$ cup toasted chopped almonds (page 87)

1 tablespoon poppy seeds

$\frac{1}{4}$ cup plus 2 tablespoons fat-free egg substitute

1 teaspoon vanilla extract

1 teaspoon almond extract

NUTRITIONAL FACTS (PER COOKIE)

Calories: 77   Carbohydrate: 14 g   Cholesterol: 0 mg
Fat: 2 g   Fiber: 1 g   Protein: 2 g   Sodium: 45 mg

DIABETIC EXCHANGES: 1 Starch, $\frac{1}{3}$ Fat

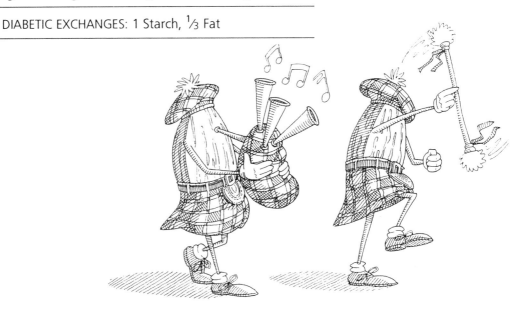

Peanut Butter-Marshmallow Treats

Yield: 20 bars

¼ cup plus 2 tablespoons creamy peanut butter

1 tablespoon water

5 cups miniature marshmallows

5 cups crisp rice cereal

1. Coat a 4-quart pot with butter-flavored cooking spray. Add the peanut butter, water, and marshmallows, cover, and cook over low heat without stirring for 3 minutes. Stir the mixture. Then continue to cook, covered, for 2 to 3 additional minutes, stirring after each minute, until the mixture is melted and smooth.

2. Remove the pot from the heat, and stir in the cereal. Coat a 9-x-13-inch baking pan with nonstick butter-flavored cooking spray, and use the back of a wooden spoon to pat the mixture evenly into the pan. (Spray the spoon with cooking spray if the mixture is sticky.)

3. Allow the mixture to cool to room temperature before cutting. Cut into 20 bars, and serve immediately, or store in an airtight container in single layers separated by sheets of waxed paper.

NUTRITIONAL FACTS (PER BAR)

Calories: 92   Carbohydrate: 16 g   Cholesterol: 0 mg
Fat: 2.4 g   Fiber: 0.5 g   Protein: 1.8 g   Sodium: 80 mg

DIABETIC EXCHANGES: 1 Starch, ½ Fat

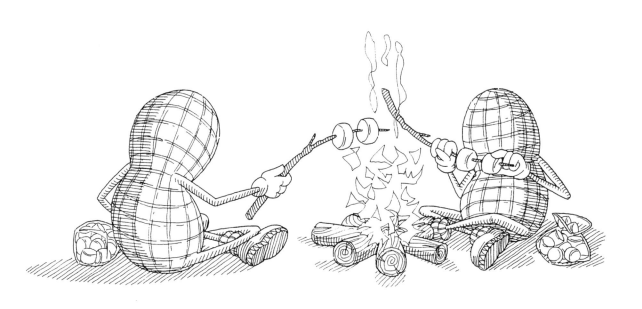

6

Refreshing Frozen Desserts

Cool and refreshing, frozen desserts are everyone's favorite treat on a sizzling summer day. But don't limit these icy confections to the summer months. Elegant and surprisingly simple to make, frozen desserts are perfect for year-round entertaining. And since they must be prepared in advance, and can then be kept in the freezer for several days, these toothsome temptations are a real boon to the busy cook.

The star ingredients in this chapter's frozen delights make these treats as healthful as they are delicious. Ripe fruits and fruit juices provide a bounty of nutrients, as well as great flavor and natural sweetness. And nonfat dairy products—including sugar-free nonfat yogurts, nonfat milk, nonfat ricotta cheese, and ready-made nonfat and low-fat ice creams—provide a significant amount of calcium, but little or no fat. Frozen desserts made from these ingredients are easily substituted for part of the fruit and milk in your meal with little or no sacrifice in nutrition.

As for sugar, these recipes contain considerably less than most traditional recipes do. In many cases, fruits, fruit juices, and juice concentrates provide a pleasing amount of natural sweetness, which is then enhanced with small amounts of artificial sweetener or sugar. In other cases, no-sugar-added ice creams are used to make inventive ice cream treats. The result? Light and refreshing sorbets and fruit whips, fruity ices, festive parfaits, and a variety of other cool confections, all made with a minimum of sugar and a maximum of important nutrients.

So whether you are looking for a simple frozen fruit pop to take the heat out of a sultry afternoon, a creamy frozen yogurt for an evening snack, or a show-stopping sorbet, parfait, or pie to impress even the most discriminating guest, you need look no further. These temptingly sweet treats will prove, once and for all, that healthful does not mean boring, and that even easy-to-make, good-for-you desserts can be satisfying and delicious.

Fruitful Frozen Yogurt

Yield: 6 servings

1. Place the fruit in a medium-sized bowl, and mash slightly with a fork. Add the yogurt, and stir to mix well.

2. Spoon the yogurt mixture into an 8-inch square pan. Cover the pan with aluminum foil, and place in the freezer for about 2 hours and 30 minutes, or until the outer 2-inch edge of the mixture is frozen.

3. Place the partially frozen mixture in the bowl of a food processor or electric mixer, breaking up the frozen outer edges. Process for about 2 minutes, or until light, creamy, and smooth.

4. Return the mixture to the pan, and return the pan to the freezer. Freeze for about 2 hours, or until firm.

5. About 20 minutes before serving, remove the dessert from the freezer and allow to soften slightly at room temperature. Scoop into individual serving dishes, and serve immediately.

1 cup fresh or frozen (thawed) fruit (try blueberries, strawberries, raspberries, blackberries, cherries, or peaches)

4 cups sugar-free nonfat vanilla yogurt

NUTRITIONAL FACTS (PER 1-CUP SERVING)

Calories: 105   Carbohydrate: 16 g   Cholesterol: 3 mg
Fat: 0.4 g   Fiber: 0.6 g   Protein: 10 g   Sodium: 126 mg

DIABETIC EXCHANGES: ¼ Fruit, 1 Skim Milk

Time-Saving Tip

If you own a 2-quart ice cream maker, you can use it to make Fruitful Frozen Yogurt. Simply pour the mixture made in Step 1 into the machine, and proceed as directed by the manufacturer.

Cantaloupe Sunshine Sorbet

Yield: 5 servings

1 cup orange juice, divided

1 envelope unflavored gelatin

6 cups fresh cantaloupe cubes
(about 1 large melon)

Sugar substitute equal to $\frac{1}{2}$ cup
sugar (page 19)

1. Place $\frac{1}{2}$ cup of the juice in a blender or food processor. Sprinkle the gelatin over the top, and let sit for 2 minutes to allow the gelatin to soften.

2. Place the remaining $\frac{1}{2}$ cup of juice in a small saucepan, and bring to a boil over high heat. Pour the heated juice into the blender over the gelatin mixture. Leaving the lid slightly ajar to allow steam to escape, blend for about 1 minute, or until the gelatin is completely dissolved.

3. Add the cantaloupe cubes and sugar substitute to the blender, and blend until smooth.

4. Spoon the mixture into an 8-inch square pan. Cover the pan with aluminum foil, and place in the freezer for about 2 hours and 30 minutes, or until the outer 2-inch edge of the mixture is frozen.

5. Place the partially frozen mixture in the bowl of a food processor or electric mixer, breaking up the frozen outer edges. Process for about 2 minutes, or until light, creamy, and smooth.

6. Return the mixture to the pan, and return the pan to the freezer. Freeze for about 2 hours, or until firm.

7. About 20 minutes before serving, remove the dessert from the freezer and allow to soften slightly at room temperature. Scoop into individual serving dishes, and serve immediately.

NUTRITIONAL FACTS (PER 1-CUP SERVING)

Calories: 89 Carbohydrate: 21 g Cholesterol: 0 mg
Fat: 0.6 g Fiber: 1.6 g Protein: 2 g Sodium: 18 mg

DIABETIC EXCHANGES: $1\frac{1}{2}$ Fruit

Time-Saving Tip

If you own a 2-quart ice cream maker, you can use it to make Cantaloupe Sunshine Sorbet. Simply pour the mixture made in Step 3 into the machine, and proceed as directed by the manufacturer.

Hawaiian Ice

1. Place the fruits, sugar substitute, and, if desired, the coconut extract in the bowl of a food processor, and process until smooth.

2. Spoon the fruit mixture into an 8-inch square pan. Cover the pan with aluminum foil, and place in the freezer for about 2 hours and 30 minutes, or until the outer 2-inch edge of the mixture is frozen.

3. Place the partially frozen mixture in the bowl of a food processor or electric mixer, breaking up the frozen outer edges. Process for about 2 minutes, or until light, creamy, and smooth.

4. Return the mixture to the pan, and return the pan to the freezer. Freeze for about 2 hours, or until firm.

5. About 20 minutes before serving, remove the dessert from the freezer and allow to soften slightly at room temperature. Scoop into individual serving dishes, and serve immediately.

Yield: 6 servings

4 cups diced fresh pineapple (about 1 large)

1½ cups sliced bananas (about 1½ large)

Sugar substitute equal to ½ cup sugar (page 19)

1 teaspoon coconut-flavored extract (optional)

NUTRITIONAL FACTS (PER ⅞-CUP SERVING)

Calories: 85 Carbohydrate: 22 g Cholesterol: 0 mg
Fat: 0.5 g Fiber: 2 g Protein: 2 g Sodium: 1 mg

DIABETIC EXCHANGES: 1½ Fruit

Time-Saving Tip

If you own a 2-quart ice cream maker, you can use it to make Hawaiian Ice. Simply pour the mixture made in Step 1 into the machine, and proceed as directed by the manufacturer.

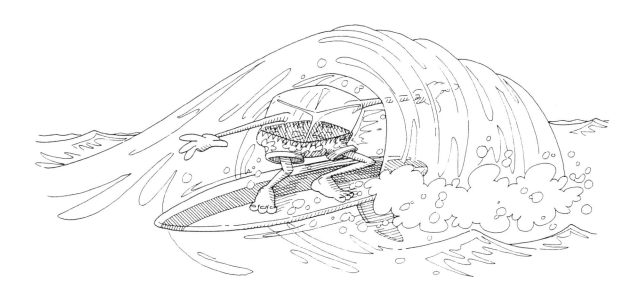

Refreshing Apricot Sorbet

Yield: 5 servings

For variety, substitute canned peaches or pears for the apricots.

2 cans (1 pound each) apricot
   halves in fruit juice, undrained

1 envelope unflavored gelatin

¼ cup sugar

Sugar substitute equal to ½ cup
   sugar (page 19)

1. Drain the apricots, reserving the juice. Set the apricots aside.

2. Place ½ cup of the reserved apricot juice in a blender or food processor. Sprinkle the gelatin over the top, and let sit for 2 minutes to allow the gelatin to soften.

3. Place another ½ cup of the juice in a small saucepan, and bring to a boil over high heat. Pour the heated juice into the blender over the gelatin mixture. Leaving the lid slightly ajar to allow steam to escape, blend for about 1 minute, or until the gelatin is completely dissolved.

4. Add the apricots, sugar, sugar substitute, and remaining juice to the blender, and blend until smooth.

5. Spoon the apricot mixture into an 8-inch square pan. Cover the pan with aluminum foil, and place in the freezer for about 2 hours and 30 minutes, or until the outer 2-inch edge of the mixture is frozen.

6. Place the partially frozen mixture in the bowl of a food processor or electric mixer, breaking up the frozen outer edges. Process for about 2 minutes, or until light, creamy, and smooth.

7. Return the mixture to the pan, and return the pan to the freezer. Freeze for about 2 hours, or until firm.

8. About 20 minutes before serving, remove the dessert from the freezer and allow to soften slightly at room temperature. Scoop into individual serving dishes, and serve immediately.

NUTRITIONAL FACTS (PER 1-CUP SERVING)
Calories: 121   Carbohydrate: 30 g   Cholesterol: 0 mg
Fat: 0.1 g   Fiber: 2.1 g   Protein: 2.3 g   Sodium: 10 mg

DIABETIC EXCHANGES: 2 Fruit

Time-Saving Tip

If you own a 2-quart ice cream maker, you can use it to make Refreshing Apricot Sorbet. Simply pour the mixture made in Step 4 into the machine, and proceed as directed by the manufacturer.

Cinnamon-Mocha Sorbet

Yield: 6 servings

1. Combine all of the ingredients in a blender or food processor, and blend at medium speed for 1 minute, or until well mixed.

2. Spoon the mixture into an 8-inch square pan. Cover the pan with aluminum foil, and place in the freezer for about 2 hours and 30 minutes, or until the outer 2-inch edge of the mixture is frozen.

3. Place the partially frozen mixture in the bowl of a food processor or electric mixer, breaking up the frozen outer edges. Process for about 2 minutes, or until light, creamy, and smooth.

4. Return the mixture to the pan, and return the pan to the freezer. Freeze for about 2 hours, or until firm.

5. About 20 minutes before serving, remove the dessert from the freezer and allow to soften slightly at room temperature. Scoop into individual serving dishes, and serve immediately.

4 cups skim or 1-percent low-fat milk

1 package (4-serving size) instant sugar-free chocolate pudding mix

$\frac{1}{2}$ cup instant nonfat dry milk powder

$\frac{1}{4}$ cup sugar

1 $\frac{1}{2}$ teaspoons instant coffee granules

$\frac{1}{2}$ teaspoon ground cinnamon

NUTRITIONAL FACTS (PER 1-CUP SERVING)

Calories: 157   Carbohydrate: 29 g   Cholesterol: 5 mg
Fat: 0.6 g   Fiber: 0 g   Protein: 9.8 g   Sodium: 376 mg

DIABETIC EXCHANGES: 1 Skim Milk, 1 Starch

Time-Saving Tip

If you own a 2-quart ice cream maker, you can use it to make Cinnamon-Mocha Sorbet. Simply pour the mixture made in Step 1 into the machine, and proceed as directed by the manufacturer.

Berry Delicious Sorbet

Yield: 6 servings

1 cup cranberry juice cocktail, divided

1 envelope unflavored gelatin

$\frac{1}{4}$ cup sugar

6 cups sliced fresh strawberries (about 8 cups whole fresh berries)

1 cup fresh or frozen (thawed) raspberries

Sugar substitute equal to $\frac{1}{2}$ cup sugar (page 19)

1. Place $\frac{1}{2}$ cup of the cranberry juice in a blender. Sprinkle the gelatin over the top, and let sit for 2 minutes to allow the gelatin to soften.

2. Place the remaining $\frac{1}{2}$ cup of juice and the sugar in a small saucepan, and bring to a boil over high heat, stirring constantly until the sugar dissolves. Pour the boiling juice mixture into the blender over the gelatin mixture. Leaving the lid slightly ajar to allow steam to escape, blend for about 1 minute, or until the gelatin is completely dissolved.

3. Add the strawberries, raspberries, and sugar substitute to the blender, and blend until smooth.

4. Spoon the mixture into an 8-inch square pan. Cover the pan with aluminum foil, and place in the freezer for about 2 hours and 30 minutes, or until the outer 2-inch edge of the mixture is frozen.

5. Place the partially frozen mixture in the bowl of a food processor or electric mixer, breaking up the frozen outer edges. Process for about 2 minutes, or until light, creamy, and smooth.

6. Return the mixture to the pan, and return the pan to the freezer. Freeze for about 2 hours, or until firm.

7. About 20 minutes before serving, remove the dessert from the freezer and allow to soften slightly at room temperature. Scoop into individual serving dishes, and serve immediately.

NUTRITIONAL FACTS (PER 1-CUP SERVING)

Calories: 128　Carbohydrate: 30 g　Cholesterol: 0 mg
Fat: 0.8 g　Fiber: 3.8 g　Protein: 2 g　Sodium: 5 mg

DIABETIC EXCHANGES: 2 Fruit

Time-Saving Tip

If you own a 2-quart ice cream maker, you can use it to make Berry Delicious Sorbet. Simply pour the mixture made in Step 3 into the machine, and proceed as directed by the manufacturer.

Maple-Apple Sorbet

Yield: 5 servings

1. Place the apple juice and apples in a $2\frac{1}{2}$-quart pot, and bring to a boil over high heat. Reduce the heat to low, cover, and simmer for 10 minutes, or until the apples are soft. Remove the pot from the heat, and allow to cool to room temperature.

2. Place the cooled apple mixture in a blender. Add the maple syrup and sugar substitute, and blend until smooth.

3. Pour the mixture into an 8-inch square pan. Cover the pan with aluminum foil, and place in the freezer for about 2 hours and 30 minutes, or until the outer 2-inch edge of the mixture is frozen.

4. Place the partially frozen mixture in the bowl of a food processor or electric mixer, breaking up the frozen outer edges. Process for about 2 minutes, or until light, creamy, and smooth.

5. Return the mixture to the pan, and return the pan to the freezer. Freeze for about 2 hours, or until firm.

6. About 20 minutes before serving, remove the dessert from the freezer and allow to soften slightly at room temperature. Scoop into individual serving dishes, and serve immediately.

3 cups unsweetened apple juice

3 cups diced peeled apples (about 4 medium)

2 tablespoons maple syrup

Sugar substitute equal to $\frac{1}{4}$ cup sugar (page 19)

NUTRITIONAL FACTS (PER $\frac{7}{8}$-CUP SERVING)

Calories: 125 Carbohydrate: 30 g Cholesterol: 0 mg
Fat: 0.4 g Fiber: 1.4 g Protein: 0.3 g Sodium: 10 mg

DIABETIC EXCHANGES: 2 Fruit

Time-Saving Tip

If you own a 2-quart ice cream maker, you can use it to make Maple-Apple Sorbet. Simply pour the mixture made in Step 2 into the machine, and proceed as directed by the manufacturer.

Sweet Cherry Spumoni

Yield: 7 servings

6 cups fresh or frozen (thawed and undrained) dark sweet pitted cherries or tart red cherries

15 ounces nonfat ricotta cheese

Sugar substitute equal to ½ cup sugar (page 19)

¼ cup dried cherries

¼ cup semi-sweet chocolate chips, coarsely chopped

¼ cup chopped toasted walnuts or almonds (page 87)

1. Place the cherries, ricotta, and sugar substitute in the bowl of a food processor or blender, and process until smooth. (Note that if you use tart red cherries, you may need to slightly increase the amount of sugar substitute.)

2. Pour the mixture into an 8-inch square pan. Cover the pan with aluminum foil, and place in the freezer for about 2 hours and 30 minutes, or until the outer 2-inch edge of the mixture is frozen.

3. Place the partially frozen mixture in the bowl of a food processor or electric mixer, breaking up the frozen outer edges. Process for about 2 minutes, or until light, creamy, and smooth. Stir in the dried cherries, chocolate chips, and nuts.

4. Return the mixture to the pan, and return the pan to the freezer. Freeze for about 2 hours, or until firm.

5. About 20 minutes before serving, remove the spumoni from the freezer and allow to soften slightly at room temperature. Scoop into individual serving dishes, and serve immediately.

NUTRITIONAL FACTS (PER 1-CUP SERVING)

Calories: 160 Carbohydrate: 21 g Cholesterol: 4 mg
Fat: 4 g Fiber: 2.5 g Protein: 9 g Sodium: 150 mg

DIABETIC EXCHANGES: 1 Fruit, ½ Skim Milk, 1 Fat

Time-Saving Tip

If you own a 2-quart ice cream maker, you can use it to make Sweet Cherry Spumoni. Simply pour the mixture made in Step 1 into the machine, and proceed as directed by the manufacturer. Add the dried cherries, chocolate chips, and nuts during the last few minutes of the creaming process.

Light Ice Cream Sandwiches

For variety, try making these sandwiches with different ice cream flavors, such as vanilla, cherry vanilla, pistachio, chocolate, peanut butter, and praline swirl.

1. Break each graham cracker in half so that you have 16 squares, each measuring $2\frac{1}{2}$ x $2\frac{1}{2}$ inches.

2. Spread $\frac{1}{4}$ cup of the ice cream over 1 square, top with another square, and gently press the crackers together. Smooth the edges of the ice cream with a knife.

3. Wrap the sandwich in plastic wrap, and place in the freezer. Repeat with the remaining ingredients to make 8 sandwiches. Freeze the sandwiches for at least 1 hour before serving.

Yield: 8 servings

8 large ($2\frac{1}{2}$-x-5-inch) reduced-fat chocolate graham crackers

2 cups nonfat no-sugar-added ice cream, any flavor, slightly softened

---

NUTRITIONAL FACTS (PER SERVING)

Calories: 100   Carbohydrate: 19 g   Cholesterol: 2 mg
Fat: 1.5 g   Fiber: 0.2 g   Protein: 3 g   Sodium: 132 mg

DIABETIC EXCHANGES: 1 Starch, $\frac{1}{4}$ Skim Milk

Almond Balls

1. Using an ice cream scoop, shape $\frac{2}{3}$-cup portions of the ice cream into 6 balls, using your hands if necessary to shape the spheres.

2. Place the almonds in a small flat dish, and roll each ball in the almonds to coat all sides. Place the balls in a covered container, and freeze for several hours or until very firm.

3. When ready to serve, place each ball in a dessert dish, and spoon 1 tablespoon of the syrup over the top. Serve immediately.

Yield: 6 servings

4 cups nonfat no-sugar-added ice cream, any flavor

$\frac{1}{2}$ cup sliced toasted almonds (page 19)

$\frac{1}{4}$ cup plus 2 tablespoons light (reduced-sugar) chocolate syrup

---

NUTRITIONAL FACTS (PER SERVING)

Calories: 178   Carbohydrate: 29 g   Cholesterol: 7 mg
Fat: 4.1 g   Fiber: 0.7 g   Protein: 7 g   Sodium: 132 mg

DIABETIC EXCHANGES: 1 Starch, 1 Skim Milk, 1 Fat

Cool Peach Melba

Yield: 6 servings

3/4 cup orange juice

3 medium peaches, peeled, halved, and pitted

3 cups nonfat no-sugar-added vanilla ice cream

SAUCE

1 tablespoon plus 1 teaspoon cornstarch

2 tablespoons sugar

1 1/4 cups fresh or frozen (unthawed) raspberries

Sugar substitute equal to 2 tablespoons sugar (page 19)

1. Place the orange juice in the bottom of a microwave or conventional steamer, and arrange the peach halves in the steamer. Cover and cook at high power or over high heat for about 4 minutes, or until the peaches are tender but not mushy. Transfer the peaches and the juice to a covered container, and refrigerate for several hours or overnight.

2. Just before serving, make the sauce by placing the cornstarch and sugar in a 1-quart saucepan. Remove 1/2 cup of juice from the container of peaches, and add it to the sugar mixture. Stir until the cornstarch dissolves.

3. Place the saucepan over medium heat, and, stirring constantly, cook for about 2 minutes, or until the mixture becomes thickened and bubbly. Add the raspberries, and bring to a second boil. Cook and stir just until the berries begin to break up. Remove the pot from the heat, and stir in the sugar substitute.

4. To assemble the desserts, place a 1/2-cup scoop of ice cream in each of 6 dessert bowls. Top each scoop with a well-drained peach half, placing the hollow side down. Top with 3 tablespoons of the warm sauce, and serve immediately.

NUTRITIONAL FACTS (PER SERVING)

Calories: 155   Carbohydrate: 35 g   Cholesterol: 5 mg
Fat: 0.4 g   Fiber: 3 g   Protein: 4.9 g   Sodium: 85 mg

DIABETIC EXCHANGES: 2 Fruit, 1/2 Milk

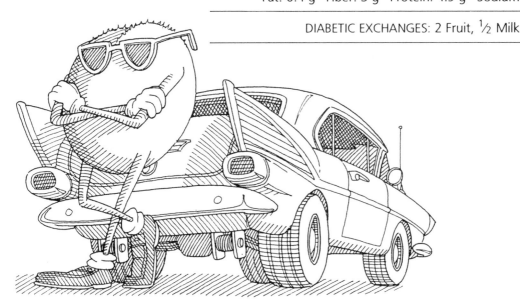

Strawberry Crunch Parfaits

1. Place the strawberries and sugar in a small bowl, and mash slightly with a fork.

2. To assemble the desserts, place 1 tablespoon of granola in the bottom of each of four 8-ounce parfait or wine glasses. Top with $\frac{1}{4}$ cup of ice cream and 1 tablespoon of the mashed strawberries. Repeat the layers, and serve immediately.

Yield: 4 servings

1 cup sliced fresh strawberries

1 tablespoon sugar

$\frac{1}{2}$ cup low-fat granola cereal

2 cups nonfat no-sugar-added vanilla ice cream

NUTRITIONAL FACTS (PER SERVING)

Calories: 143   Carbohydrate: 30 g   Cholesterol: 5 mg
Fat: 0.7 g   Fiber: 1.1 g   Protein: 5 g   Sodium: 111 mg

DIABETIC EXCHANGES: 1 Starch, 1 Fruit

Cherry Angel Parfaits

1. Cut each slice of cake into 4 portions, so that you have 8 portions of cake.

2. To assemble the desserts, crumble 1 portion of cake into the bottom of each of four 8-ounce parfait or wine glasses. Top with $\frac{1}{4}$ cup of ice cream, and 1 tablespoon of the pie filling. Repeat the layers, and serve immediately.

Yield: 4 servings

2 slices (1 ounce each) angel food cake

2 cups nonfat no-sugar-added vanilla or chocolate ice cream

$\frac{1}{2}$ cup canned light (reduced-sugar) cherry pie filling

---

NUTRITIONAL FACTS (PER SERVING)

Calories: 139   Carbohydrate: 29 g   Cholesterol: 5 mg
Fat: 0.1 g   Fiber: 0.4 g   Protein: 5 g   Sodium: 195 mg

DIABETIC EXCHANGES: 1 Starch, $\frac{1}{2}$ Fruit, $\frac{1}{2}$ Skim Milk

Island Ice Cream Delight

Yield: 4 servings

2 cups nonfat no-sugar-added
  vanilla ice cream

SAUCE

$\frac{1}{4}$ cup orange juice

1 teaspoon cornstarch

$\frac{1}{4}$ teaspoon ground nutmeg

1 tablespoon honey

1 large ripe but firm banana,
  sliced

Sugar substitute equal to 2
  tablespoons sugar (page 19)

1. To make the sauce, place the orange juice and cornstarch in a 1-quart saucepan, and stir to dissolve the cornstarch. Add the nutmeg and honey, and stir to mix well.

2. Place the saucepan over medium heat, and bring to a boil, stirring constantly. Stir for another 30 seconds, or until the mixture is thickened and bubbly. Add the bananas, and cook for another minute, or until the bananas are heated through and slightly softened. Remove the pot from the heat, and stir in the sugar substitute.

3. To assemble the desserts, place a $\frac{1}{2}$-cup scoop of ice cream into each of four 8-ounce balloon wine glasses. Top each serving with $2\frac{1}{2}$ tablespoons of the warm sauce, and serve immediately.

NUTRITIONAL FACTS (PER SERVING)

Calories: 132 Carbohydrate: 29 g Cholesterol: 5 mg
Fat: 0.2 g Fiber: 0.6 g Protein: 4.4 g Sodium: 86 mg

DIABETIC EXCHANGES: $1\frac{1}{2}$ Fruit, $\frac{1}{2}$ Skim Milk

---

Sensational Strawberry Pops

Yield: 10 pops

4 cups sliced fresh strawberries

$\frac{1}{2}$ cup frozen white grape juice
  concentrate or frozen
  cranberry juice concentrate,
  thawed

1. Place the strawberries and juice concentrate in the bowl of a food processor or blender, and process until smooth. (If preferred, leave the mixture slightly chunky.)

2. Spoon the mixture into ten $2\frac{1}{2}$-ounce popsicle molds or $2\frac{1}{2}$-ounce paper cups. If using molds, insert the sticks and freeze for several hours, or until firm. If using paper cups, let the pops partially freeze before inserting a popsicle stick in the center of each.

3. When ready to serve, remove from the freezer, and let stand at room temperature for 3 minutes before unmolding the pops. Serve immediately.

NUTRITIONAL FACTS (PER POP)

Calories: 43 Carbohydrate: 10 g Cholesterol: 0 mg
Fat: 0.2 g Fiber: 1 g Protein: 0.4 g Sodium: 1 mg

DIABETIC EXCHANGES: $\frac{2}{3}$ Fruit

Frozen Yogurt Fruit Pops

Yield: 10 pops

1. Place the fruit and yogurt in the bowl of a food processor or blender, and process until smooth. (If preferred, leave the mixture slightly chunky.)

2. Spoon the mixture into ten $2\frac{1}{2}$-ounce popsicle molds or $2\frac{1}{2}$-ounce paper cups. If using molds, insert the sticks and freeze for several hours, or until firm. If using paper cups, let the pops partially freeze before inserting a popsicle stick in the center of each.

3. When ready to serve, remove from the freezer, and let stand at room temperature for 3 minutes before unmolding the pops. Serve immediately.

2 cups very ripe, sweet fruit (try blueberries, strawberries, peaches, nectarines, or bananas)

2 cups sugar-free nonfat vanilla yogurt

NUTRITIONAL FACTS (PER POP)

Calories: 43 Carbohydrate: 8 g Cholesterol: 1 mg
Fat: 0.2 g Fiber: 0.8 g Protein: 3 g Sodium: 39 mg

DIABETIC EXCHANGES: $\frac{1}{4}$ Skim Milk, $\frac{1}{3}$ Fruit

---

Berries and Cream Cake

Yield: 12 servings

1. With a serrated knife, cut a $1\frac{1}{2}$-inch-deep channel in the top of the angel food cake, leaving $\frac{3}{8}$ inch of cake intact on either side of the channel. Spoon the ice cream evenly into the hollowed-out section of the cake. Wrap the cake in plastic wrap, and freeze for at least 3 hours or until serving time.

2. When ready to serve, remove the cake from the freezer, and remove and discard the plastic wrap. Place the cake in the center of a 12-inch round platter.

3. Combine the strawberries and blueberries in a large bowl, and toss to mix well. Arrange $1\frac{1}{2}$ cups of the fruit mixture on top of the cake, over the ice cream. Arrange the remaining fruit around the base of the cake. Slice and serve immediately.

1 angel food cake (1 pound)

2 cups nonfat no-sugar-added vanilla ice cream, slightly softened

3 cups sliced fresh strawberries

$1\frac{1}{2}$ cups fresh blueberries

NUTRITIONAL FACTS (PER SERVING)

Calories: 135 Carbohydrate: 30 Cholesterol: 2 mg
Fat: 0.5 g Fiber: 1.6 g Protein: 3.7 g Sodium: 278 mg

DIABETIC EXCHANGES: 1 Starch, 1 Fruit

Frozen Mocha Pie

Yield: 8 servings

¼ cup light (reduced-sugar) chocolate syrup

2 tablespoons coffee liqueur

2 cups light whipped topping

4 ounces ladyfingers (about 16 whole cookies)

3 cups nonfat no-sugar-added chocolate ice cream, slightly softened

1 teaspoon cocoa powder

1. To make the syrup, combine the chocolate syrup and liqueur in a small bowl, and stir to mix well. Set aside.

2. To make the topping, place the whipped topping in a medium-sized bowl, and gently fold in 1 tablespoon of the chocolate syrup mixture. Set aside.

3. To assemble the pie, first split each of the ladyfingers in half lengthwise. (Most ladyfingers come presplit.) Line the bottom and sides of a 9-inch deep-dish pie pan with about two-thirds of the ladyfinger halves, arranging them split side-up. Drizzle half of the chocolate syrup mixture over the ladyfingers that line the bottom of the pan.

4. Spread the ice cream over the ladyfingers. Then top with the remaining ladyfingers, this time arranging them split side-down.

5. Drizzle the remaining chocolate syrup mixture over the ladyfingers layer. Then spread the whipping topping mixture over the syrup, swirling the topping.

6. Cover the pie with aluminum foil or plastic wrap, and freeze for several hours or overnight. When ready to serve, sprinkle the cocoa over the top of the pie. Cut the pie into wedges, place the wedges on individual serving plates, and let sit at room temperature for 5 minutes before serving.

NUTRITIONAL FACTS (PER SERVING)
Calories: 164 Carbohydrate: 34 Cholesterol: 30 mg
Fat: 2.7 g Fiber: 0.2 g Protein: 4.2 g Sodium: 103 mg

DIABETIC EXCHANGES: 1½ Starch, ½ Skim Milk, ½ Fat

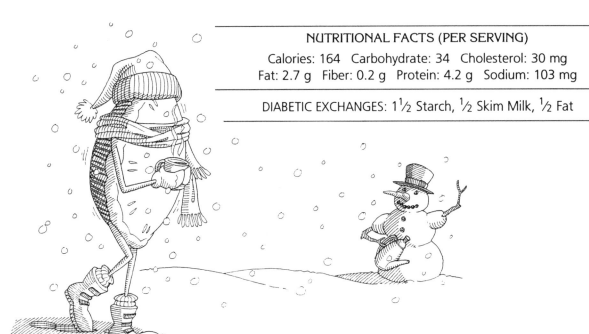

7

Crisps, Cobblers, and Other Fabulous Fruit Desserts

When you want a dessert full of down-home goodness, think cobblers and crisps. With their fruit fillings, cobblers and crisps are naturally sweet and delicious. And when made properly, these treats contain surprisingly little sugar and fat. In fact, the fillings of the desserts presented in this chapter are sweetened mostly by the natural sugar present in the fruit itself. The inclusion of fruit juices and dried fruits also adds natural sweetness. Then flavorings like cinnamon and nutmeg further enhance sweetness, reducing the need for sugar and sugar substitutes.

Of course, in most traditional fruit-based desserts, the biggest source of fat is the topping. It's not unusual for the cinnamon-flavored crumbs atop an apple crisp to contain as much as a full stick of butter—as well as a cup of brown sugar! As you will see, by using the right ingredients, it's easy to greatly reduce both fat and sugar without sacrificing the flavors and textures you love. In this chapter, the crisp and crumble toppings combine naturally sweet grain products like whole grain oats and oat bran with a variety of other wholesome ingredients, such as toasted wheat germ, nuts, fruit juice concentrate, cinnamon, and ginger. These toppings are so full of natural crunch, spice, and sweetness that only very small amounts of sweeteners are needed. Cobbler crusts are made from unbleached and whole grain flours, and moistened with nonfat buttermilk and other nonfat dairy products. Full of down-home goodness, these delightfully sweet toppings are low in both fat and sugar.

When creating desserts with fresh fruits, do be sure to use very ripe sweet produce, as this will reduce the need for added sugar and insure a flavorful result. But don't think that cobblers and crisps can be made only during the summer months, when fresh fruits are most bountiful! A wide variety of tempting desserts are possible even on the coldest winter day, as these recipes take advantage of fresh fruits from every season of the year, as well as frozen fruits and fruits canned in juice. Served hot from the oven, these heart-warming treats will provide your family with old-fashioned comfort all year long.

Mixed Fruit Crisp

1. To make the filling, place the apples, pears, plums, raisins or dried cranberries, and sugar substitute in a large bowl, and toss to mix well. Coat a 9-inch pie pan with nonstick cooking spray, and spread the fruit mixture evenly in the pan. Set aside.

2. To make the topping, break up the graham crackers, place them in a blender or food processor, and process into crumbs. Measure the crumbs. There should be ¾ cup. (Adjust the amount if necessary.)

3. Place the crumbs, brown sugar, walnuts, cinnamon, and ginger in a small bowl, and stir to mix well. Using a pastry cutter or 2 knives, cut in the margarine or butter until the mixture is moist and crumbly. Sprinkle the topping over the filling.

4. Bake uncovered at 375°F for 35 minutes, or until the filling is bubbly and the topping is golden brown. Cover loosely with aluminum foil during the last few minutes of baking if the topping starts to brown too quickly. Serve warm or at room temperature.

Yield: 8 servings

FILLING

2 medium apples, peeled and thinly sliced

2 medium pears, peeled and cut into ¾-inch chunks

2 medium unpeeled red plums, cut into ¾-inch slices

¼ cup dark raisins or dried cranberries

Sugar substitute equal to 2 tablespoons sugar (page 19)

TOPPING

4½ large (2½-x-5-inch) low-fat graham crackers

¼ cup light brown sugar

2 tablespoons finely ground walnuts

¼ teaspoon ground cinnamon

¼ teaspoon ground ginger

2 tablespoons reduced-fat margarine or light butter, cut into pieces

---

NUTRITIONAL FACTS (PER SERVING)

Calories: 150   Carbohydrate: 30 g   Cholesterol: 0 mg
Fat: 3.5 g   Fiber: 2.5 g   Protein: 1.7 g   Sodium: 87 mg

DIABETIC EXCHANGES: 1 Starch, 1 Fruit, ¾ Fat

Summer Fruit Crisp

Yield: 6 servings

FILLING

4 cups sliced peeled peaches or nectarines (about 6 medium)

1 cup fresh or frozen (unthawed) blueberries

1 tablespoon cornstarch

Sugar substitute equal to ¼ cup sugar (page 19)

TOPPING

¼ cup plus 2 tablespoons quick-cooking oats or oat bran

3 tablespoons whole wheat pastry flour

¼ cup light brown sugar

3 tablespoons honey-toasted wheat germ

¼ teaspoon ground cinnamon

1 tablespoon plus 2 teaspoons reduced-fat margarine or light butter, cut into pieces

2 teaspoons frozen (thawed) orange juice concentrate

1. To make the filling, place the peaches or nectarines, blueberries, cornstarch, and sugar substitute in a large bowl, and toss gently to mix well. Coat a 9-inch pie pan with nonstick cooking spray, and spread the mixture evenly in the pan. Set aside.

2. To make the topping, place the oats or oat bran, flour, brown sugar, wheat germ, and cinnamon in a small bowl, and stir to mix well. Using a pastry cutter or 2 knives, cut in the margarine or butter until the mixture is crumbly. Stir in the juice concentrate until the mixture is moist and crumbly. Sprinkle the topping over the filling.

3. Bake uncovered at 375°F for 35 to 40 minutes, or until the filling is bubbly and the topping is golden brown. Cover loosely with aluminum foil during the last few minutes of baking if the topping starts to brown too quickly. Serve warm or at room temperature.

NUTRITIONAL FACTS (PER SERVING)

Calories: 152   Carbohydrate: 32 g   Cholesterol: 0 mg
Fat: 2.5 g   Fiber: 3.9 g   Protein: 3 g   Sodium: 18 mg

DIABETIC EXCHANGES: 1 Starch, 1 Fruit, ½ Fat

Plum Delicious Crisp

Yield: 8 servings

FILLING

6 cups sliced unpeeled ripe red plums (about 8 medium-large)

2 tablespoons light brown sugar

1. To make the filling, place the plums and brown sugar in a large bowl, and toss to mix well. Coat an 8-inch square baking dish with nonstick cooking spray, and spread the mixture evenly in the pan. Set aside.

2. To make the topping, place the oats, flour, sugar, walnuts, and cinnamon or ginger in a medium-sized bowl, and stir to mix well. Add the juice concentrate, and stir until the mixture is moist and crumbly. Sprinkle the topping over the filling.

3. Bake uncovered at 375°F for 35 minutes, or until the plums are tender and the topping is golden brown. Cover loosely with aluminum foil during the last 10 to 15 minutes of baking if the topping starts to brown too quickly. Serve warm.

TOPPING

½ cup quick-cooking oats

¼ cup whole wheat pastry flour

¼ cup light brown sugar

¼ cup chopped walnuts

½ teaspoon ground cinnamon or ginger

2 tablespoons frozen (thawed) apple juice concentrate

NUTRITIONAL FACTS (PER SERVING)

Calories: 157 Carbohydrate: 31 g Cholesterol: 0 mg
Fat: 3.4 g Fiber: 3.6 g Protein: 3.3 g Sodium: 4 mg

DIABETIC EXCHANGES: 1 Starch, 1 Fruit, ⅔ Fat

Hawaiian Pineapple Crisp

1. To make the filling, place the pineapple, cornstarch, nutmeg, and sugar substitute in a large bowl, and toss to mix well. Coat a 9-inch pie pan with nonstick cooking spray, and spread the mixture evenly in the pan. Set aside.

2. To make the topping, place the oats, flour, and brown sugar in a medium-sized bowl, and stir to mix well. Using a pastry cutter or 2 knives, cut in the margarine or butter until the mixture is moist and crumbly. Stir in the coconut. Sprinkle the topping over the filling.

3. Bake uncovered at 375°F for 35 minutes, or until the filling is bubbly and the topping is golden brown. Cover loosely with aluminum foil during the last few minutes of baking if the topping starts to brown too quickly. Serve warm.

Yield: 6 servings

FILLING

4 cups fresh pineapple, cut into bite-sized pieces (about 1 medium)

2 teaspoons cornstarch

¼ teaspoon ground nutmeg

Sugar substitute equal to ¼ cup sugar (page 19)

TOPPING

½ cup quick-cooking oats

¼ cup whole wheat pastry flour

¼ cup light brown sugar

2 tablespoons reduced-fat margarine or light butter, cut into pieces

¼ cup shredded sweetened coconut

NUTRITIONAL FACTS (PER SERVING)

Calories: 149 Carbohydrate: 29 g Cholesterol: 0 mg
Fat: 3.6 Fiber: 2.7 g Protein: 2.3 g Sodium: 28 mg

DIABETIC EXCHANGES: 1 Starch, 1 Fruit, ¾ Fat

Apple-Raisin Crisp

Yield: 6 servings

FILLING

5 cups sliced peeled apples (about 7 medium)

3 tablespoons dark raisins

Brown sugar substitute equal to 2 tablespoons brown sugar (page 19)

1 teaspoon butter-flavored extract

TOPPING

¼ cup barley nugget cereal

¼ cup light brown sugar

3 tablespoons whole wheat pastry flour

2 tablespoons honey-toasted wheat germ

¼ teaspoon ground cinnamon

⅛ teaspoon ground nutmeg

1 tablespoon frozen (thawed) apple juice concentrate

1. To make the filling, place the apples, raisins, sugar substitute, and extract in a large bowl, and toss to mix well. Coat a 9-inch pie pan with nonstick cooking spray, and spread the mixture evenly in the pan. Set aside.

2. To make the topping, place the cereal, brown sugar, flour, wheat germ, cinnamon, and nutmeg in a small bowl, and stir to mix well. Add the juice concentrate, and stir until the mixture is moist and crumbly. Sprinkle the topping over the filling.

3. Bake uncovered at 375°F for 35 minutes, or until the filling is bubbly and the topping is golden brown. Cover loosely with aluminum foil during the last few minutes of baking if the topping starts to brown too quickly. Serve warm or at room temperature.

NUTRITIONAL FACTS (PER SERVING)

Calories: 133   Carbohydrate: 32 g   Cholesterol: 0 mg
Fat: 0.6 g   Fiber: 2.9 g   Protein: 1.9 g   Sodium: 36 mg

DIABETIC EXCHANGES: 1 Starch, 1 Fruit

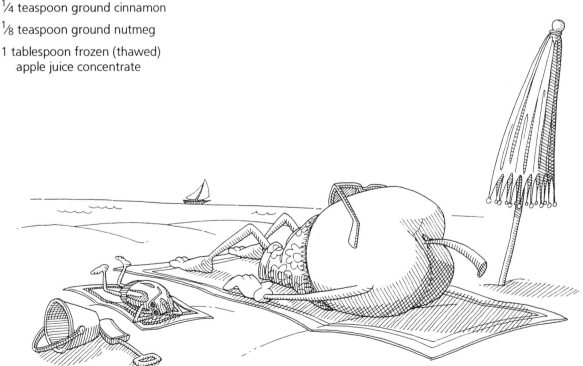

Cocoa Fruit Crisp

Yield: 8 servings

1. To make the filling, place the pears, dried cherries, and sugar substitute in a large bowl, and toss to mix well. Coat a 9-inch pie pan with nonstick cooking spray, and spread the mixture evenly in the pan. Set aside.

2. To make the topping, combine the oats, brown sugar, cocoa, and flour in a small bowl, and stir to mix well. Using a pastry cutter or 2 knives, cut in the margarine or butter until the mixture is moist and crumbly. Stir in the walnuts, and sprinkle the topping over the filling.

3. Bake uncovered at 375°F for 35 minutes, or until the filling is bubbly and the topping is golden brown. Cover loosely with aluminum foil during the last few minutes of baking if the topping starts to brown too quickly. Serve warm or at room temperature.

FILLING

6 cups peeled pears, cut into ¾-inch chunks (about 6 medium)

¼ cup dried cherries

Sugar substitute equal to ¼ cup sugar (page 19)

TOPPING

⅓ cup quick-cooking oats

⅓ cup light brown sugar

2 tablespoons Dutch processed cocoa powder

2 tablespoons whole wheat pastry flour

2 tablespoons reduced-fat margarine or light butter, cut into pieces

3 tablespoons chopped walnuts

NUTRITIONAL FACTS (PER SERVING)

Calories: 163 Carbohydrate: 32 g Cholesterol: 0 mg
Fat: 4 g Fiber: 4.3 g Protein: 2.4 g Sodium: 15 mg

DIABETIC EXCHANGES: 1 Starch, 1 Fruit, 1 Fat

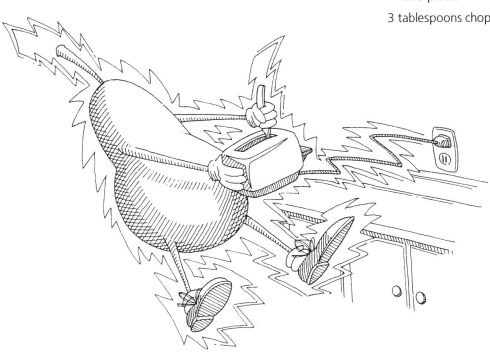

Peach-Almond Crisp

Yield: 8 servings

FILLING

5 cups sliced peeled peaches
(about 7 medium)

¼ cup golden raisins or chopped
dates

Sugar substitute equal to ¼ cup
sugar (page 19)

TOPPING

2 cups oat flake-and-almond cereal

¼ cup light brown sugar

¼ teaspoon ground ginger

¼ teaspoon ground nutmeg

2 tablespoons reduced-fat
margarine or light butter, cut
into pieces

¼ cup sliced almonds

1. To make the filling, place the peaches, raisins or dates, and sugar substitute in a large bowl, and toss to mix well. Coat an 8-inch square baking dish with nonstick cooking spray, and spread the fruit mixture evenly in the pan. Set aside.

2. To make the topping, place the cereal in a blender and process into crumbs. Measure the crumbs. There should be ¾ cup plus 2 tablespoons. (Adjust the amount if necessary.)

3. Place the crumbs, brown sugar, ginger, and nutmeg in a small bowl, and stir to mix well. Using a pastry cutter or 2 knives, cut in the margarine or butter until the mixture is moist and crumbly. Stir in the almonds, and sprinkle the topping over the filling.

4. Bake uncovered at 375°F for 35 minutes, or until the filling is bubbly and the topping is golden brown. Cover loosely with aluminum foil during the last few minutes of baking if the topping starts to brown too quickly. Serve warm or at room temperature.

NUTRITIONAL FACTS (PER SERVING)

Calories: 166 Carbohydrate: 32 g Cholesterol: 0 mg
Fat: 3.2 g Fiber: 2.9 g Protein: 2.9 g Sodium: 67 mg

DIABETIC EXCHANGES: 1 Starch, 1 Fruit, ½ Fat

California Crumble

Yield: 6 servings

FILLING

1 can (1 pound) sliced peaches
packed in juice, undrained

1 can (1 pound) apricot halves
packed in juice, undrained

¼ cup chopped pitted prunes or
dates

1. To make the filling, drain the peaches and apricots, reserving 2 tablespoons of the juice from either fruit. Place the peaches, apricots, reserved juice, and prunes or dates in a large bowl, and toss to mix well. Coat a 9-inch pie pan with nonstick cooking spray, and spread the mixture evenly in the pan. Set aside.

2. To make the topping, combine the oat bran, wheat germ, flour, brown sugar, and cinnamon in a small bowl, and stir to mix well. Using a pastry cutter or 2 knives, cut in the margarine or butter until the mixture is moist and crumbly. Sprinkle the topping over the filling.

3. Bake uncovered at 375°F for 30 minutes, or until the filling is bubbly and the topping is golden brown. Cover loosely with aluminum foil during the last few minutes of baking if the topping starts to brown too quickly. Serve warm or at room temperature.

TOPPING

¼ cup oat bran

¼ cup toasted wheat germ

2 tablespoons whole wheat flour

⅓ cup light brown sugar

½ teaspoon ground cinnamon

2 tablespoons reduced-fat margarine or light butter, cut into pieces

---

NUTRITIONAL FACTS (PER SERVING)

Calories: 148 Carbohydrate: 31 g Cholesterol: 0 mg
Fat: 3.1 g Fiber: 4 g Protein: 3.7 g Sodium: 21 mg

DIABETIC EXCHANGES: 1 Starch, 1 Fruit, ½ Fat

Cherry-Apple Crisp

1. To make the filling, place the apples, cherries, dried cherries, and sugar substitute in a large bowl, and toss to mix well. Coat an 8-inch square baking dish with nonstick cooking spray, and spread the mixture evenly in the pan. Set aside.

2. To make the topping, break up the graham crackers, place them in a blender, and process into crumbs. Measure the crumbs. There should be ¾ cup. (Adjust the amount if necessary.)

3. Place the crumbs, brown sugar, and cinnamon in a small bowl, and stir to mix well. Using a pastry cutter or 2 knives, cut in the margarine or butter until the mixture is moist and crumbly. Stir in the pecans, and sprinkle the topping over the filling.

4. Bake uncovered at 375°F for 35 minutes, or until the filling is bubbly and the topping is golden brown. Cover loosely with aluminum foil during the last few minutes of baking if the topping starts to brown too quickly. Serve warm or at room temperature.

Yield: 8 servings

FILLING

5 cups sliced peeled apples (about 7 medium)

1 cup pitted fresh or frozen (thawed) cherries

⅓ cup dried cherries

Sugar substitute equal to 3 tablespoons sugar (page 19)

TOPPING

4½ large (2½-x-5-inch) low-fat graham crackers

¼ cup light brown sugar

½ teaspoon ground cinnamon

2 tablespoons reduced-fat margarine or light butter, cut into pieces

¼ cup finely chopped pecans

NUTRITIONAL FACTS (PER SERVING)

Calories: 164 Carbohydrate: 30 g Cholesterol: 0 mg
Fat: 4.8 g Fiber: 2.3 g Protein: 1.5 g Sodium: 86 mg

DIABETIC EXCHANGES: 1 Starch, 1 Fruit, 1 Fat

Plum Batter Bake

Yield: 8 servings

FILLING

3$\frac{1}{2}$ cups sliced unpeeled ripe red plums (about 5 medium-large)

$\frac{1}{4}$ teaspoon ground cinnamon

2 tablespoons maple syrup

TOPPING

$\frac{3}{4}$ cup whole wheat pastry flour

3 tablespoons sugar

1 teaspoon baking powder

$\frac{1}{4}$ teaspoon baking soda

$\frac{3}{4}$ cup nonfat or low-fat buttermilk

2 egg whites

1 teaspoon vanilla extract

2 tablespoons powdered sugar

For variety, substitute sliced peeled peaches, apples, or pears for the plums.

1. To make the filling, place the plums and cinnamon in a medium-sized bowl, and toss to mix well. Coat an 8-inch square baking dish with nonstick cooking spray, and spread the mixture evenly in the pan. Drizzle the maple syrup over the top.

2. Cover the pan with aluminum foil, and bake at 425°F for 15 minutes, or until the plums begin to soften.

3. To make the topping, place all of the topping ingredients in a blender or food processor, and blend for about 45 seconds, or until smooth. Pour the topping over the hot fruit, and bake uncovered for 15 additional minutes, or until the topping is lightly browned.

4. Remove the dish from the oven, and sift the powdered sugar over the top. Allow to cool for 10 minutes before serving warm.

NUTRITIONAL FACTS (PER SERVING)

Calories: 139 Carbohydrate: 30 g Cholesterol: 1 mg
Fat: 0.9 Fiber: 2 g Protein: 3.5 g Sodium: 123 mg

DIABETIC EXCHANGES: 1 Starch, 1 Fruit

Cherry Batter Bake

Yield: 8 servings

FILLING

3 tablespoons sugar

1 tablespoon plus 1 teaspoon cornstarch

1 package (12 ounces) frozen (thawed) pitted sweet cherries or pitted tart red cherries

3 tablespoons orange juice

For variety, substitute blueberries or blackberries for the cherries.

1. To make the filling, place the sugar and cornstarch in a 1$\frac{1}{2}$-quart pot, and stir to mix well. Drain the juice from the thawed cherries, and add the juice to the pot, setting the cherries aside. Stir until the cornstarch is dissolved. Stir in the orange juice.

2. Place the pot over medium heat, and cook, stirring constantly, until the mixture is thickened and bubbly. Add the cherries, and cook, still stirring, for another minute, or until the mixture is heated through. (Note that if you use tart cherries, you will need to add sugar substitute equal to $\frac{1}{4}$ cup sugar at this point.) If the mixture seems too thick, add a little more orange juice.

3. Coat an 8-inch square baking dish with nonstick cooking spray, and pour the hot cherry mixture into the pan. Set aside.

4. To make the topping, place all of the topping ingredients in a blender or food processor, and blend for about 45 seconds, or until smooth. Pour the topping over the hot fruit, and bake uncovered at 425°F for 15 minutes, or until the topping is lightly browned.

5. Remove the dish from the oven, and sift the powdered sugar over the top. Allow to cool for 10 minutes before serving warm.

TOPPING

¾ cup unbleached flour

3 tablespoons sugar

1½ teaspoons baking powder

¾ cup evaporated skimmed milk

2 egg whites

1 teaspoon vanilla extract

½ teaspoon almond extract

2 tablespoons powdered sugar

NUTRITIONAL FACTS (PER SERVING)

Calories: 144 Carbohydrate: 31 g Cholesterol: 1 mg
Fat: 0.3 g Fiber: 1.3 g Protein: 4.5 g Sodium: 110 mg

DIABETIC EXCHANGES: 1 Starch, 1 Fruit

Apple-Strawberry Cobbler

Yield: 8 servings

1. To make the filling, place the apples, strawberries, and cornstarch in a large bowl, and toss to mix well. Add the apple juice and sugar substitute, and toss to mix well.

2. Coat a 2-quart casserole dish with nonstick cooking spray, and spread the mixture evenly in the dish. Cover the dish with aluminum foil, and bake at 375°F for 30 minutes, or until the mixture is hot and bubbly.

3. To make the topping, place the flour, oats, sugar, baking powder, and baking soda in a medium-sized bowl, and stir to mix well. Add just enough of the buttermilk to make a moderately stiff dough, stirring just until the dry ingredients are moistened. Drop rounded tablespoons of batter onto the hot fruit filling to make 8 biscuits.

4. Bake uncovered at 375°F for 18 to 20 minutes, or until the biscuits are lightly browned. Remove the dish from the oven, and allow to cool for 10 minutes before serving warm.

FILLING

5 cups coarsely chopped peeled apples (about 7 medium)

2 cups coarsely chopped fresh strawberries

1 tablespoon cornstarch

3 tablespoons apple juice

Sugar substitute equal to ½ cup sugar (page 19)

BISCUIT TOPPING

1 cup unbleached flour

⅓ cup quick-cooking oats

⅓ cup sugar

1 teaspoon baking powder

¼ teaspoon baking soda

½ cup plus 2 tablespoons nonfat buttermilk

NUTRITIONAL FACTS (PER SERVING)

Calories: 165 Carbohydrate: 38 g Cholesterol: 0 mg
Fat: 0.9 g Fiber: 2.7 g Protein: 3 g Sodium: 104 mg

DIABETIC EXCHANGES: 1 Starch, 1½ Fruit

Biscuit-Topped Blueberry Cobbler

Yield: 8 servings

6 cups fresh or frozen (partially thawed) blueberries

2 tablespoons cornstarch

Sugar substitute equal to ¼ cup plus 2 tablespoons sugar (page 19)

2 tablespoons frozen (thawed) orange juice concentrate

BISCUIT TOPPING

1 cup unbleached flour

⅓ cup oat bran

⅓ cup sugar

1 teaspoon baking powder

¼ teaspoon baking soda

½ cup plus 2 tablespoons nonfat buttermilk

1. To make the filling, place the berries, cornstarch, sugar substitute, and juice concentrate in a large bowl, and stir to mix well.

2. Coat a 2-quart casserole dish with nonstick cooking spray, and spread the mixture evenly in the dish. Cover the dish with aluminum foil, and bake at 375°F for 30 to 40 minutes, or until the mixture is hot and bubbly.

3. To make the topping, place the flour, oat bran, sugar, baking powder, and baking soda in a medium-sized bowl, and stir to mix well. Add just enough of the buttermilk to form a moderately stiff batter, stirring just until the dry ingredients are moistened. Drop heaping tablespoonfuls of the batter onto the hot fruit filling to make 8 biscuits.

4. Bake uncovered at 375°F for 18 to 20 minutes, or until the biscuits are lightly browned. Remove the dish from the oven, and allow to cool for 10 minutes before serving warm.

NUTRITIONAL FACTS (PER SERVING)

Calories: 182   Carbohydrate: 43 g   Cholesterol: 0 mg
Fat: 0.9 g   Fiber: 4.1 g   Protein: 3.8 g   Sodium: 112 mg

DIABETIC EXCHANGES: 1 Starch, 2 Fruit

Cinnamon Apple Cobbler

Yield: 9 servings

FILLING

2 teaspoons cornstarch

½ cup plus 1 tablespoon unsweetened apple juice, divided

6 cups sliced peeled apples (about 9 medium)

¾ teaspoon ground cinnamon

Brown sugar substitute equal to ¼ cup brown sugar (page 19)

1. To make the filling, place the cornstarch and 1 tablespoon of the apple juice in a small bowl, and stir to mix well. Set aside.

2. Place the apples, the remaining ½ cup of apple juice, and the cinnamon in a 3-quart pot, and bring to a boil over high heat. Reduce the heat to medium-low, cover, and cook, stirring occasionally, for about 8 minutes, or until the apples begin to soften. Stir the cornstarch mixture, and add it to the pot. Cook and stir uncovered for another minute, or until the mixture thickens. Remove the pot from the heat, and stir in the sugar substitute.

3. Coat a 2-quart casserole dish with nonstick cooking spray, and spread the hot mixture evenly in the dish.

4. To make the topping, place the flour, sugar, baking powder, and baking soda in a medium-sized bowl, and stir to mix well. Add the buttermilk and egg white, and stir just until the dry ingredients are moistened. Spread the batter evenly over the hot fruit.

5. Bake uncovered at 400°F for 20 minutes, or until the cobbler is bubbly around the edges and the topping is golden brown. Remove the dish from the oven, and allow to cool for 10 minutes before serving warm.

TOPPING

³⁄₄ cup plus 2 tablespoons whole wheat pastry flour or unbleached flour

¹⁄₄ cup plus 2 tablespoons sugar

1 teaspoon baking powder

¹⁄₄ teaspoon baking soda

³⁄₄ cup nonfat or low-fat buttermilk

1 egg white, lightly beaten

NUTRITIONAL FACTS (PER SERVING)

Calories: 134 Carbohydrate: 31 g Cholesterol: 0 mg
Fat: 0.6 g Fiber: 2.8 g Protein: 2.8 g Sodium: 104 mg

DIABETIC EXCHANGES: 1 Starch, 1 Fruit

Cranberry Pear Crumble

1. To make the filling, place the pears, cranberries, brown sugar, and sugar substitute in a large bowl, and toss to mix well. Coat a 9-inch pie pan with nonstick cooking spray, and spread the fruit mixture evenly in the pan. Set aside.

2. To make the topping, place the oat bran, flour, brown sugar, and cinnamon in a medium-sized bowl, and stir to mix well. Using a pastry cutter or 2 knives, cut in the margarine or butter until the mixture is crumbly. Sprinkle the topping over the filling.

3. Bake uncovered at 375°F for 35 minutes, or until the filling is bubbly and the topping is golden brown. Cover loosely with aluminum foil during the last few minutes of baking if the topping starts to brown too quickly. Serve warm or at room temperature.

Yield: 8 servings

FILLING

5 cups diced peeled pears (about 5 medium)

¹⁄₂ cup coarsely chopped fresh or frozen (unthawed) cranberries

2 tablespoons light brown sugar

Sugar substitute equal to 3 tablespoons sugar (page 19)

TOPPING

¹⁄₃ cup oat bran

¹⁄₄ cup whole wheat pastry flour

¹⁄₃ cup light brown sugar

¹⁄₄ teaspoon ground cinnamon

2 tablespoons reduced-fat margarine or light butter, cut into pieces

---

NUTRITIONAL FACTS (PER SERVING)

Calories: 130 Carbohydrate: 30 g Cholesterol: 0 mg
Fat: 2.3 g Fiber: 3.7 g Protein: 1.6 g Sodium: 16 mg

DIABETIC EXCHANGES: 1 Starch, 1 Fruit, ¹⁄₂ Fat

Mini Blackberry Cobblers

Yield: 6 servings

FILLING

4 cups fresh or frozen (thawed) blackberries

1 tablespoon cornstarch

1 tablespoon frozen (thawed) apple juice concentrate

Sugar substitute equal to $\frac{1}{3}$ cup sugar (page 19)

CRUST

$\frac{1}{2}$ cup unbleached flour

$\frac{1}{2}$ cup whole wheat pastry flour

1 tablespoon sugar

$\frac{1}{2}$ teaspoon baking powder

3 tablespoons chilled reduced-fat margarine or light butter, cut into pieces

3 tablespoons skim milk

GLAZE

1 egg white, beaten, or 2 tablespoons fat-free egg substitute

$1\frac{1}{2}$ teaspoons sugar

1. To make the filling, place the blackberries, cornstarch, juice concentrate, and sugar substitute in a large bowl, and toss to mix well. Coat six 6-ounce custard cups with nonstick cooking spray, and divide the mixture evenly among the cups. Set aside.

2. To make the crust, place the flours, sugar, and baking powder in a medium-sized bowl, and stir to mix well. Using a pastry cutter or 2 knives, cut in the margarine or butter until the mixture resembles coarse crumbs. Add just enough of the milk to make a stiff dough, stirring just until the dough holds together and forms a ball.

3. Shape the dough into 6 balls. Using a rolling pin and working on a lightly floured surface, roll each ball into a 4-inch circle, and lay 1 crust over the fruit filling in each cup. Pinch the edges of each circle to make a decorative edge.

4. To glaze the crusts, brush them lightly with the egg white, and sprinkle $\frac{1}{4}$ teaspoon of sugar over the top. Using a sharp knife, cut 4 slits in the center of each crust to allow steam to escape during baking.

5. Place the cups on a baking sheet, and bake at 375°F for 30 minutes, or until the filling is bubbly and the crusts are golden brown. Remove the cobblers from the oven, and allow to cool for at least 10 minutes before serving warm.

NUTRITIONAL FACTS (PER SERVING)

Calories: 174   Carbohydrate: 33 g   Cholesterol: 0 mg
Fat: 3.6 g   Fiber: 5.8 g   Protein: 4 g   Sodium: 70 mg

DIABETIC EXCHANGES: 1 Starch, 1 Fruit, $\frac{3}{4}$ Fat

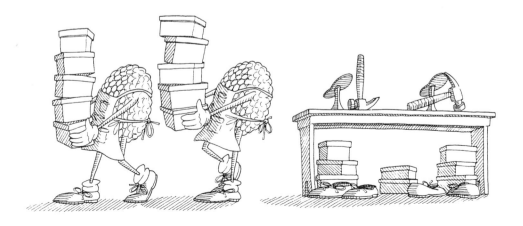

Spiced Pear Cobbler

For variety, substitute canned peaches for the pears.

Yield: 8 servings

1. To make the filling, drain the pears, reserving $\frac{3}{4}$ cup plus 2 tablespoons of the juice. Cut the pears into chunks and set aside.

2. Place the cornstarch, cinnamon, nutmeg, and 2 tablespoons of the reserved juice in a small dish. Stir until smooth, and set aside.

3. Pour the remaining $\frac{3}{4}$ cup of reserved juice into a 2-quart pot, and bring to a boil over medium heat. Slowly stir in the cornstarch mixture, and cook, still stirring, for a minute or 2, or until the mixture is thickened and bubbly. Add the pears to the pot, and cook and stir for an additional minute or 2, or until the mixture returns to a boil. Remove the pot from the heat, stir in the sugar substitute, and cover to keep warm.

4. To make the topping, combine the flour, oat bran, sugar, and baking powder in a medium-sized bowl, and stir to mix well. Add the egg substitute and yogurt, and stir just until the dry ingredients are moistened.

5. Coat a 2-quart casserole dish with nonstick cooking spray, and spread the warm fruit mixture evenly in the dish. Spread the batter topping over the fruit, and bake at 400°F for 25 minutes, or until the filling is bubbly and the topping is golden brown. Remove the dish from the oven, and allow to cool for at least 10 minutes before serving warm.

FILLING

2 cans (1 pound each) pear halves in juice, undrained

1 tablespoon cornstarch

$\frac{1}{2}$ teaspoon ground cinnamon

$\frac{1}{4}$ teaspoon ground nutmeg

Sugar substitute equal to $\frac{1}{4}$ cup plus 2 tablespoons sugar (page 19)

TOPPING

$\frac{1}{2}$ cup unbleached flour

$\frac{1}{4}$ cup oat bran

$\frac{1}{4}$ cup plus 2 tablespoons sugar

$1\frac{1}{4}$ teaspoons baking powder

$\frac{1}{4}$ cup fat-free egg substitute

$\frac{1}{4}$ cup plain nonfat yogurt

NUTRITIONAL FACTS (PER SERVING)

Calories: 137 Carbohydrate: 32 g Cholesterol: 0 mg
Fat: 0.4 g Fiber: 2.3 g Protein: 3 g Sodium: 80 mg

DIABETIC EXCHANGES: 1 Starch, 1 Fruit

Three-Fruit Cobbler

Yield: 8 servings

FILLING

1 can (1 pound) apricot halves in juice, undrained

1 can (1 pound) sliced peaches in juice, undrained

1 can (10 ounces) mandarin orange segments in juice, undrained

1 tablespoon plus 1½ teaspoons cornstarch

½ teaspoon ground cinnamon

2 tablespoons sugar

Sugar substitute equal to ⅓ cup sugar (page 19)

CRUST

½ cup oat bran

½ cup unbleached flour

1 teaspoon baking powder

3 tablespoons chilled reduced-fat margarine or light butter, cut into pieces

2–3 tablespoons skim milk

GLAZE

2 teaspoons fat-free egg substitute

2 teaspoons water

1 tablespoon sugar

1. To make the filling, drain the apricots, peaches, and oranges, reserving ¾ cup of the mixed juice. Cut the apricot halves in half, and combine them with the peaches and oranges in a medium-sized bowl. Set aside.

2. Place the cornstarch, cinnamon, and 2 tablespoons of the reserved juice in a small dish, and stir until smooth. Set aside.

3. Pour the remaining reserved juice into a 2-quart pot. Add the sugar, and bring to a boil over medium heat. Reduce the heat to low, and slowly stir in the cornstarch mixture. Cook, still stirring, for another minute, or until the mixture is thickened and bubbly.

4. Add the fruit to the juice mixture, and stir until the fruit is coated with the glaze. Remove the pot from the heat, and stir in the sugar substitute. Coat a 10-inch pie pan with nonstick cooking spray, and spread the filling evenly in the pan. Set aside.

5. To make the crust, place the oat bran, flour, and baking powder in a medium-sized bowl, and stir to mix well. Using a pastry cutter or 2 knives, cut in the margarine or butter until the mixture resembles coarse crumbs. Stir in just enough of the milk to make a stiff dough that leaves the sides of the bowl and forms a ball.

6. Turn the dough onto a floured surface, and, using a rolling pin, roll into an 11-inch circle. Use a knife or pizza wheel to cut the circle into ½-inch strips.

7. Arrange half of the crust strips over the filling, spacing them ½-inch apart. Arrange the remaining strips over the filling in the opposite direction to form a lattice top. Trim any edges to make the dough conform to the shape of the pan.

8. To glaze the crust, combine the egg substitute and water in a small dish, and brush over the crust. Sprinkle the tablespoon of sugar over the crust.

9. Bake at 375°F for 30 minutes, or until the filling is bubbly and the crust is lightly browned. Remove the dish from the oven, and allow to cool for at least 10 minutes. Serve warm or at room temperature.

NUTRITIONAL FACTS (PER SERVING)

Calories: 140   Carbohydrate: 30 g   Cholesterol: 0 mg
Fat: 2.9 g   Fiber: 2.7 g   Protein: 3 g   Sodium: 71 mg

DIABETIC EXCHANGES: 1 Starch, 1 Fruit, ½ Fat

Cranberry Baked Apples

1. To make the syrup, place 1 tablespoon of the juice, the cornstarch, and the cinnamon in a 1-quart pot, and stir to mix well. Stir in the remaining juice, and place the pot over medium heat. Cook and stir for about 2 minutes, or until the mixture comes to a boil and thickens slightly. Remove the pot from the heat, and stir in the sugar substitute. Set aside.

2. Core the apples, starting at the stem end, but do not cut through the opposite end. Peel the top third of each apple.

3. Coat an 8-inch square pan with nonstick cooking spray, and arrange the apples in the pan. Place the nuts and the cranberries or raisins in a small dish, and toss to mix well. Spoon 1½ tablespoons of the nut mixture into the cavity of each apple. Drizzle the syrup over and around the apples.

4. Cover the pan with aluminum foil, and bake at 350°F for 30 minutes. Remove the foil, and spoon some of the hot syrup from the pan over the apples. Bake uncovered for 10 additional minutes, or until the apples are tender. Transfer the apples to serving dishes, and spoon some of the syrup over the top. Serve hot.

Yield: 4 servings

4 medium-sized apples

¼ cup chopped walnuts

2 tablespoons chopped dried cranberries or dark raisins

SYRUP

¾ cup plus 2 tablespoons cranberry juice cocktail

2 teaspoons cornstarch

¼ teaspoon ground cinnamon

Brown sugar substitute equal to ¼ cup brown sugar (page 19)

NUTRITIONAL FACTS (PER SERVING)

Calories: 171   Carbohydrate: 33 g   Cholesterol: 0 mg
Fat: 5 g   Fiber: 3.3 g   Protein: 2.3 g   Sodium: 2 mg

DIABETIC EXCHANGES: 2 Fruit, 1 Fat

Ginger Baked Peaches

Yield: 6 servings

3 large peaches (8 ounces each)

3 tablespoons orange juice

FILLING

¼ cup barley nugget cereal

¼ cup light brown sugar

3 tablespoons whole wheat pastry flour

¼ teaspoon ground ginger

¼ teaspoon ground cinnamon

1 tablespoon plus ½ teaspoon frozen (thawed) orange juice concentrate

TOPPING

¼ cup sugar-free nonfat vanilla yogurt

⅛ teaspoon ground ginger

½ cup light whipped topping

1. To make the filling, place the cereal, brown sugar, flour, ginger, and cinnamon in a small bowl, and stir to mix well. Add the juice concentrate, and stir just until the mixture is moist and crumbly. Set aside.

2. Peel the peaches. Then cut each in half lengthwise, and remove the pit. Cut a thin slice off the bottom of each peach half so that it will sit upright. Place a rounded tablespoon of the filling in the cavity of each peach half, mounding it slightly.

3. Pour the orange juice into the bottom of a 9-inch square pan, and arrange the peaches in the pan. Bake uncovered at 375°F for 25 to 30 minutes, or until the peaches are tender and the filling is golden brown. Cover the peaches loosely with aluminum foil during the last few minutes of baking if the filling starts to brown too quickly.

4. While the peaches are baking, prepare the topping. Place the yogurt and ginger in a small bowl, and stir to mix well. Gently fold in the whipped topping. Serve the peaches warm, topping each peach half with 2 tablespoons of the topping.

NUTRITIONAL FACTS (PER SERVING)

Calories: 113   Carbohydrate: 26 g   Cholesterol: 0 mg
Fat: 0.9 g   Fiber: 2.6 g   Protein: 2.4 g   Sodium: 45 mg

DIABETIC EXCHANGES: ¾ Starch, 1 Fruit

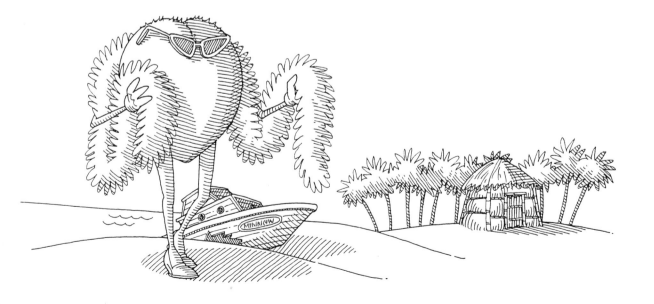

8

Delightful Dessert Breads

Quick breads and other sweet breads are among the most versatile of desserts. Served plain, with low-fat cream cheese, or with a glass of low-fat milk, they can double as nutritious breakfast breads or as great mid-morning and late-night snacks. Filled with fruits and nuts and topped with a temptingly sweet glaze, they can provide a glorious finale to even the most festive of dinners.

Like cakes and most other baked goods, though, sweet breads do need some sugar if they are to have a pleasing texture. Without at least some sugar, breads have a coarse, tough consistency, and do not brown properly. In fact, most traditional quick bread recipes contain close to a full cup of sugar per loaf! But, as you will see, sweet and delicious breads can be made with half the usual sugar. How? Sweet grains like oats, oat bran, and whole wheat pastry flour, and naturally sweet fruits and juices allow you to add relatively small amounts of sweetener, and still enjoy truly luscious results.

Unlike many reduced-sugar recipes, which add extra fat to produce a pleasing texture, the recipes in this chapter contain no butter, margarine, oil, or other shortening at all. Instead, these recipes skillfully combine ingredients like whole grain flours, oat bran, and rolled oats with fruit purées, juices, nonfat buttermilk, and other healthful fat substitutes. The result? Moist and delicious breads made with no butter, oil, or other fats, and with a lot less sugar than you'll find in most traditional recipes.

So whether you're looking for a festive fruit and nut loaf for holiday gift giving, a warm fruit-filled yeast bread to serve with coffee, or a whole wheat banana-nut bread to accompany a late-night glass of milk, you need look no further. In this chapter you will find a wide variety of sweet and delightful loaves that are special enough to fit any occasion, but healthful enough to merit a regular place in your diet.

Whole Wheat Banana-Nut Bread

1. Place the flour, sugar, baking powder, baking soda, and nutmeg in a large bowl, and stir to mix well. Add the banana, and stir just until the dry ingredients are moistened. Fold in the walnuts.

2. Coat an 8-x-4-inch loaf pan with nonstick cooking spray. Spread the mixture evenly in the pan, and bake at 325°F for about 55 minutes, or just until a toothpick inserted in the center of the loaf comes out clean.

3. Remove the bread from the oven, and let sit for 10 minutes. Invert the loaf onto a wire rack, turn right side up, and cool to room temperature. Wrap the loaf in aluminum foil or plastic wrap, and let sit overnight before slicing and serving. (Overnight storage will give the loaf a softer, moister crust.)

Yield: 16 slices

2 cups whole wheat pastry flour

½ cup sugar

1 teaspoon baking powder

1 teaspoon baking soda

½ teaspoon ground nutmeg

2 cups mashed very ripe banana (about 4 large)

½ cup chopped walnuts

NUTRITIONAL FACTS (PER SLICE)

Calories: 125 Carbohydrate: 24 g Cholesterol: 0 mg
Fat: 2.6 g Fiber: 2.6 g Protein: 3.3 g Sodium: 102 mg

DIABETIC EXCHANGES: 1 Starch, ½ Fruit, ½ Fat

Applesauce-Oatmeal Bread

1. Place the flour, oats, sugar, baking powder, baking soda, and cinnamon in a large bowl, and stir to mix well. Add the applesauce and vanilla extract, and stir just until the dry ingredients are moistened. Fold in the raisins and walnuts.

2. Coat an 8-x-4-inch loaf pan with nonstick cooking spray. Spread the mixture in the pan, and bake at 325°F for 45 minutes, or just until a toothpick inserted in the center of the loaf comes out clean.

3. Remove the bread from the oven, and let sit for 10 minutes. Invert the loaf onto a wire rack, turn right side up, and cool to room temperature. Wrap the loaf in aluminum foil or plastic wrap, and let sit overnight before slicing and serving. (Overnight storage will give the loaf a softer, moister crust.)

Yield: 16 slices

1½ cups whole wheat pastry flour

¾ cup quick-cooking oats

½ cup sugar

1 teaspoon baking powder

1 teaspoon baking soda

¾ teaspoon ground cinnamon

1½ cups unsweetened applesauce

1 teaspoon vanilla extract

⅓ cup dark raisins

⅓ cup chopped walnuts

NUTRITIONAL FACTS (PER SLICE)

Calories: 103 Carbohydrate: 20 g Cholesterol: 0 mg
Fat: 1.9 g Fiber: 2 g Protein: 2.9 g Sodium: 103 mg

DIABETIC EXCHANGES: 1 Starch, ⅓ Fruit, ⅓ Fat

Cocoa Banana Bread

Yield: 16 slices

1²⁄₃ cups whole wheat pastry flour

¹⁄₂ cup sugar

¹⁄₃ cup Dutch processed cocoa
    powder

1 teaspoon baking powder

1 teaspoon baking soda

2 cups mashed very ripe banana
    (about 4 large)

1¹⁄₂ teaspoons vanilla extract

¹⁄₃ cup chopped walnuts

¹⁄₃ cup semi-sweet chocolate chips

1. Place the flour, sugar, cocoa, baking powder, and baking soda in a large bowl, and stir to mix well. Add the banana and vanilla extract, and stir just until the dry ingredients are moistened. Fold in the walnuts and chocolate chips.

2. Coat an 8-x-4-inch loaf pan with nonstick cooking spray. Spread the mixture evenly in the pan, and bake at 325°F for about 55 minutes, or just until a wooden toothpick inserted in the center of the loaf comes out clean.

3. Remove the bread from the oven, and let sit for 10 minutes. Invert the loaf onto a wire rack, turn right side up, and cool to room temperature. Wrap the loaf in aluminum foil or plastic wrap, and let sit overnight before slicing and serving. (Overnight storage will give the loaf a softer, moister crust.)

NUTRITIONAL FACTS (PER SLICE)

Calories: 129 Carbohydrate: 25 g Cholesterol: 0 mg
Fat: 3 g Fiber: 3 g Protein: 3.1 g Sodium: 103 mg

DIABETIC EXCHANGES: 1 Starch, ¹⁄₂ Fruit, ¹⁄₂ Fat

Baking Festive Round Loaves

Any quick bread recipe can be used to make festive round loaves by baking the batter in cans instead of loaf pans. These loaves can then be wrapped in colored plastic wrap, tied on top with a ribbon, and given as gifts during the holiday season or at any time of the year.

Simply coat three or four 1-pound food cans with nonstick cooking spray, and divide the batter evenly among the cans, filling each half full. Bake at 300°F for about 45 minutes, or just until a wooden toothpick inserted in the center of a loaf comes out clean. Cool the bread in the cans for 10 minutes, remove the loaves from the cans, and cool completely before wrapping.

A word of caution is in order regarding the cans used to make these loaves. When choosing cans for baking, be sure to avoid those that have been lead-soldered. Lead is a toxic metal that can leach into foods during baking. Food cans produced in this country do not contain lead solder, as the United States canning industry eliminated this process in 1991. Some labels even state that the can is lead-free. Imported foods, however, may still be packaged in soldered cans.

To be safe, avoid baking bread in all cans with pronounced seams—a sign of possible lead soldering—and in all imported food cans. You will then be sure that your festive breads are as healthy as they are delicious.

Pumpkin Spice Bread

1. Place the flour, oats, sugar, baking soda, and pumpkin pie spice in a large bowl, and stir to mix well. Add the pumpkin and the juice, and stir just until the dry ingredients are moistened. Fold in the dried fruit and nuts.

2. Coat four 1-pound cans with nonstick cooking spray. Divide the batter evenly among the cans, and bake at 300°F for about 50 minutes, or just until a wooden toothpick inserted in the center of a loaf comes out clean.

3. Remove the bread from the oven, and let sit for 10 minutes. Invert the loaves onto a wire rack, turn right side up, and cool to room temperature. Wrap the loaves in aluminum foil or plastic wrap, and let sit overnight before slicing and serving. (Overnight storage will give the loaves a softer, moister crust.)

Yield: 32 slices

2¼ cups whole wheat pastry flour

1 cup quick-cooking oats

¾ cup sugar

1 teaspoon baking soda

1 tablespoon pumpkin pie spice

1 cup mashed cooked or canned pumpkin

1½ cups apple or orange juice

½ cup dried cranberries, dark raisins, or chopped dates

½ cup chopped walnuts or pecans

NUTRITIONAL FACTS (PER SLICE)

Calories: 84   Carbohydrate: 17 g   Cholesterol: 0 mg
Fat: 1.4 g   Fiber: 1.7 g   Protein: 2.2 g   Sodium: 41 mg

DIABETIC EXCHANGES: 1 Starch

Fruit and Nut Bread

1. Place the flour, sugar, baking powder, and baking soda in a large bowl, and stir to mix well. Add the buttermilk and vanilla extract, and stir just until the dry ingredients are moistened. Fold in the fruits and nuts.

2. Coat four 1-pound cans with nonstick cooking spray. Divide the batter among the cans, and bake at 300°F for 40 minutes, or just until a wooden toothpick inserted in the center of a loaf comes out clean.

3. Remove the bread from the oven, and let sit for 10 minutes. Invert the loaves onto a wire rack, turn right side up, and cool to room temperature. Wrap the loaves in aluminum foil or plastic wrap, and let sit overnight before slicing and serving. (Overnight storage will give the loaves a softer, moister crust.)

Yield: 28 slices

2 cups whole wheat pastry flour

½ cup sugar

1 teaspoon baking powder

1 teaspoon baking soda

1¼ cups nonfat or low-fat buttermilk

2 teaspoons vanilla extract

¼ cup dried cherries or cranberries

¼ cup chopped dried pineapple

¼ cup dark raisins

¼ cup golden raisins

⅔ cup chopped walnuts, pecans, or almonds

NUTRITIONAL FACTS (PER SLICE)

Calories: 83   Carbohydrate: 15 g   Cholesterol: 0 mg
Fat: 1.9 g   Fiber: 1.4 g   Protein: 2.4 g   Sodium: 70 mg

DIABETIC EXCHANGES: ½ Starch, ½ Fruit, ⅓ Fat

Fresh Pear Bread

Yield: 16 slices

2 cups whole wheat pastry flour

½ cup sugar

1 teaspoon baking powder

1 teaspoon baking soda

¼ teaspoon ground nutmeg

¼ teaspoon ground cinnamon

¾ cup pear nectar

1 teaspoon vanilla extract

1⅓ cups finely chopped peeled pear (about 1½ medium)

⅓ cup dried currants or dark raisins

1. Place the flour, sugar, baking powder, baking soda, nutmeg, and cinnamon in a large bowl, and stir to mix well. Add the nectar, vanilla extract, and pears, and stir just until the dry ingredients are moistened. Fold in the currants or raisins.

2. Coat an 8-x-4-inch loaf pan with nonstick cooking spray. Spread the mixture evenly in the pan, and bake at 325°F for about 45 minutes, or just until a wooden toothpick inserted in the center of the loaf comes out clean.

3. Remove the bread from the oven, and let sit for 10 minutes. Invert the loaf onto a wire rack, turn right side up, and cool to room temperature. Wrap the loaf in aluminum foil or plastic wrap, and let sit overnight before slicing and serving. (Overnight storage will give the loaf a softer, moister crust.)

NUTRITIONAL FACTS (PER SLICE)

Calories: 100 Carbohydrate: 24 g Cholesterol: 0 mg
Fat: 0.3 g Fiber: 2.5 g Protein: 2.2 g Sodium: 103 mg

DIABETIC EXCHANGES: 1 Starch, ½ Fruit

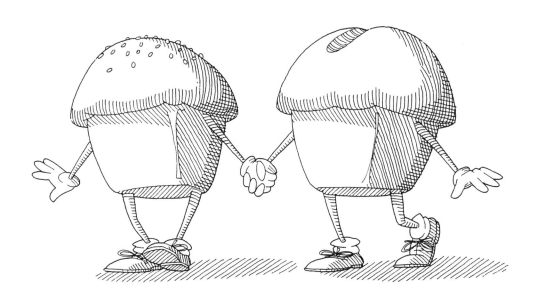

Orange Date-Nut Bread

1. Place the oats and orange juice in a small bowl, and stir to mix well. Set aside for 5 minutes.

2. Place the flour, sugar, baking powder, baking soda, and orange rind in a large bowl, and stir to mix well. Add the orange juice mixture and the evaporated milk, and stir just until the dry ingredients are moistened. Fold in the dates and nuts.

3. Coat an 8-x-4-inch loaf pan with nonstick cooking spray. Spread the mixture evenly in the pan, and bake at 325°F for about 45 minutes, or just until a wooden toothpick inserted in the center of the loaf comes out clean.

4. Remove the bread from the oven, and let sit for 10 minutes. Invert the loaf onto a wire rack, turn right side up, and cool to room temperature. Wrap the loaf in aluminum foil or plastic wrap, and let sit overnight before slicing and serving. (Overnight storage will give the loaf a softer, moister crust.)

Yield: 16 slices

¾ cup quick-cooking oats

1 cup orange juice

1½ cups whole wheat pastry flour

½ cup sugar

1 teaspoon baking powder

1 teaspoon baking soda

1 teaspoon dried grated orange rind

¼ cup evaporated skimmed milk

½ cup chopped dates

⅓ cup chopped pecans or walnuts

NUTRITIONAL FACTS (PER SLICE)
Calories: 118   Carbohydrate: 23 g   Cholesterol: 0 mg
Fat: 2 g   Fiber: 2.3 g   Protein: 3.3 g   Sodium: 107 mg

DIABETIC EXCHANGES: 1 Starch, ½ Fruit, ⅓ Fat

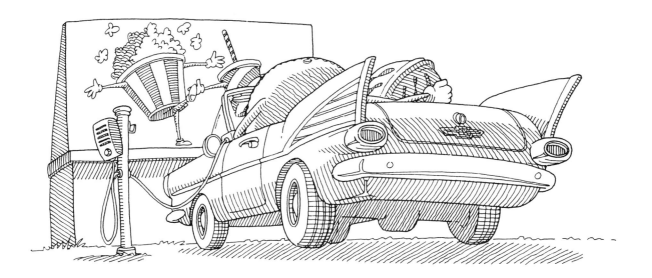

Strawberry-Oat Bran Bread

Yield: 24 slices

3 cups sliced fresh strawberries

1¾ cups whole wheat pastry flour

1 cup oat bran

¾ cup sugar

¾ teaspoon baking soda

¼ cup evaporated skimmed milk

1½ teaspoons vanilla extract

½ cup chopped almonds or
   walnuts

1.   Place the strawberries in a blender or food processor, and process until you have a smooth purée. Measure the purée. There should be 1½ cups. (Adjust the amount if necessary.) Set aside.

2.   Place the flour, oat bran, sugar, and baking soda in a large bowl, and stir to mix well. Add the puréed strawberries, evaporated milk, and vanilla extract, and stir just until the dry ingredients are moistened. Fold in the almonds or walnuts.

3.   Coat three 1-pound cans with nonstick cooking spray. Divide the batter evenly among the cans, and bake at 300°F for about 50 minutes, or just until a wooden toothpick inserted in the center of a loaf comes out clean.

4.   Remove the bread from the oven, and let sit for 10 minutes. Invert the loaves onto a wire rack, turn right side up, and cool to room temperature. Wrap in aluminum foil or plastic wrap, and let sit overnight before slicing and serving. (Overnight storage will give the loaves a softer, moister crust.)

NUTRITIONAL FACTS (PER SLICE)

Calories: 87   Carbohydrate: 17 g   Cholesterol: 0 mg
Fat: 1.9 g   Fiber: 2.2 g   Protein: 2.7 g   Sodium: 43 mg

DIABETIC EXCHANGES: 1 Starch, ⅓ Fat

Southern Sweet Potato Bread

1. Place the flour, cornmeal, baking soda, and orange rind in a large bowl, and stir to mix well. Add the sweet potato, orange juice, and molasses or honey, and stir just until the dry ingredients are moistened. Fold in the pecans.

2. Coat four 1-pound cans with nonstick cooking spray. Divide the batter evenly among the cans, and bake at 300°F for about 45 minutes, or just until a wooden toothpick inserted in the center of a loaf comes out clean.

3. Remove the bread from the oven, and let sit for 10 minutes. Invert the loaves onto a wire rack, turn right side up, and cool to room temperature. Wrap the loaves in aluminum foil or plastic wrap, and let sit overnight before slicing and serving. (Overnight storage will give the loaves a softer, moister crust.)

Yield: 32 slices

2¼ cups whole wheat pastry flour

1 cup whole grain cornmeal

1 teaspoon baking soda

1 teaspoon dried grated orange rind

1 cup mashed cooked sweet potato

1¼ cups orange juice

¾ cup molasses or honey

1 cup chopped toasted pecans (page 87)

NUTRITIONAL FACTS (PER SLICE)

Calories: 93　Carbohydrate: 16 g　Cholesterol: 0 mg
Fat: 2.4 g　Fiber: 1.8 g　Protein: 2.1 g　Sodium: 50 mg

DIABETIC EXCHANGES: 1 Starch, ½ Fat

Cinnamon-Apple Chop Bread

1. To make the dough, place ¾ cup of the flour and all of the oats, sugar, yeast, and salt in a large bowl, and stir to mix well. Set aside.

2. Place the milk in a small saucepan, and heat until very warm (125°F to 130°F). Add the milk to the flour mixture, and stir for 1 minute. Stir in enough of the remaining flour, 2 tablespoons at a time, to form a soft dough.

3. Sprinkle 2 tablespoons of the remaining flour over a flat surface, and turn the dough onto the surface. Knead the dough for 5 minutes, gradually adding just enough of the remaining flour to form a smooth, satiny ball.

4. Coat a large bowl with nonstick cooking spray, and place the dough in the bowl. Cover the bowl with a clean kitchen towel, and let rise in a warm place for about 35 minutes, or until doubled in size.

Yield: 8 wedges

DOUGH

1½ cups bread flour

¼ cup plus 2 tablespoons quick-cooking oats

2 tablespoons sugar

2 teaspoons Rapid Rise yeast

¼ teaspoon salt

½ cup plus 2 tablespoons skim milk

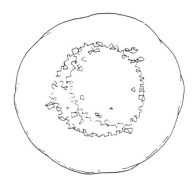

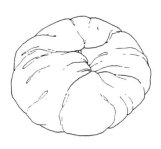

a. Pile the filling on the circle of dough.

b. Draw the dough up and around the filling.

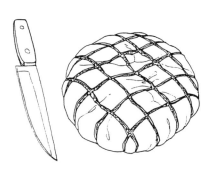

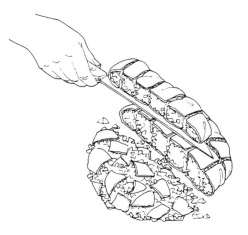

c. Slice the dough-wrapped mound 5 times in each direction.

d. Use a knife to gently mix the dough and the filling.

Making Cinnamon-Apple Chop Bread.

Time-Saving Tip

To make the dough for Cinnamon-Apple Chop Bread in a bread machine, simply place all of the dough ingredients except for $\frac{1}{4}$ cup of the bread flour in the machine's bread pan. (Do not heat any of the liquids.) Turn the machine to the "rise," "dough," "manual," or equivalent setting so the machine will mix, knead, and let the dough rise once.

Check the dough about 5 minutes after the machine has started. If the dough seems too sticky, add more of the remaining flour, a tablespoon at a time. When the dough is ready, remove it from the machine and proceed to shape, fill, and bake it as directed in the recipe.

5. To make the filling, place the apples, sugar, and cinnamon in a small bowl, and toss to mix well. Add the nuts, and toss to mix well. Set aside.

6. Place the dough on a large floured cutting board, and pat it into a 10-inch circle. Pile the apple mixture on top of the dough, and draw the dough up and around the apple mixture so that the edges of the dough meet in the middle, completely covering the apple filling. Flatten the dough into an 8-inch circle.

7. Using a large sharp knife, slice the dough-wrapped mound 5 times in one direction, cutting all the way through to the board. Then slice 5 times in the other direction to form pieces of dough that are about $1\frac{1}{2}$ inches square. Use the knife to gently mix the dough and apple mixture by lifting the dough and apple mixture from the bottom and piling it back on the top.

8. Coat a baking sheet with nonstick cooking spray, and gently mound the dough onto the sheet. Using your hands, gently shape the dough into an 8-inch circle, making sure that most of the apple mixture is touching pieces of dough. (This will insure that the bread holds together as it bakes.)

9. Cover the loaf with a clean kitchen towel, and let rise in a warm place for about 30 minutes, or until nearly doubled in size. Brush the top lightly with skim milk, and bake at 350°F for about 23 minutes, or until the bread is light golden brown and puffy. Remove the bread from the oven, and allow to cool for 3 to 5 minutes.

10. To make the glaze, place all of the glaze ingredients in a small bowl, and stir until smooth. Drizzle the glaze over the warm loaf, and immediately cut into wedges and serve.

FILLING

$1\frac{3}{4}$ cups chopped peeled apples (about $2\frac{1}{2}$ medium)

1 tablespoon sugar

1 teaspoon ground cinnamon

$\frac{1}{4}$ cup chopped walnuts or pecans

GLAZE

$\frac{1}{3}$ cup powdered sugar

$1\frac{1}{2}$ teaspoons skim milk

$\frac{1}{4}$ teaspoon vanilla extract

NUTRITIONAL FACTS (PER SERVING)

Calories: 164   Carbohydrate: 31 g   Cholesterol: 0 mg
Fat: 2.7 g   Fiber: 1.7 g   Protein: 4.3 g   Sodium: 77 mg

DIABETIC EXCHANGES: 1 Starch, 1 Fruit, $\frac{1}{2}$ Fat

Festive Fruit Bread

Yield: 12 servings

3 tablespoons warm water (105°F–115°F)

2 teaspoons Rapid Rise yeast

3 tablespoons plus 1 teaspoon sugar, divided

1¾ cups bread flour

½ cup oat bran or quick-cooking oats

1 teaspoon dried grated orange rind

¼ teaspoon ground nutmeg or cardamom

¼ teaspoon salt

½ cup plain nonfat yogurt, brought to room temperature

1 egg white

¼ cup golden raisins

¼ cup dark raisins

¼ cup dried cranberries

¼ cup chopped almonds

2 teaspoons skim milk

2 tablespoons powdered sugar

1. Place the water, yeast, and 1 teaspoon of the sugar in a small bowl, and stir to dissolve the yeast. Set aside.

2. Place the remaining 3 tablespoons of sugar, ¾ cup of the flour, and all of the oat bran or oats, orange rind, nutmeg or cardamom, and salt in a large bowl. Stir to mix well.

3. Add the yeast mixture, yogurt, and egg white to the flour mixture, and stir for 1 minute.

4. Add 2 tablespoons of the remaining flour to the dough, and stir to mix. Stir in enough of the remaining flour, 2 tablespoons at a time, to form a stiff dough. Stir in the dried fruits and almonds.

5. Sprinkle 2 tablespoons of the remaining flour onto a flat surface, and turn the dough onto the surface. Knead for 5 minutes, gradually adding enough of the remaining flour to form a satiny ball.

6. Coat a large bowl with nonstick cooking spray, and place the dough in the bowl. Cover the bowl with a clean kitchen towel, and let rise in a warm place for about 1 hour, or until doubled in size.

7. When the dough has risen, place it on a lightly floured surface, and divide it into 3 portions. Using your hands, roll each piece into a 22-inch rope. Braid the ropes together, and bring the ends around to form a ring. Pinch the ends together to seal.

8. Coat a 9-inch round cake pan with nonstick cooking spray, and place the ring in the pan. Cover with a clean kitchen towel, and let rise in a warm place for about 1 hour, or until doubled in size.

9. Brush the top of the ring with the 2 teaspoons of skim milk, and bake at 350°F for about 23 minutes, or until lightly browned.

Time-Saving Tip

To make the dough for Festive Fruit Bread in a bread machine, simply place all of the dough ingredients, except for ¼ cup of the bread flour and the dried fruits and nuts, in the machine's bread pan. (Do not heat any of the liquids.) Turn the machine to the "raisin bread," "fruit and nut," or equivalent setting so that the machine will mix, knead, and let the dough rise once.

Check the dough about 5 minutes after the machine has started. If the dough seems too sticky, add more of the remaining flour, a tablespoon at a time. Add the fruits and nuts when the machine so indicates. When the dough is ready, remove it from the machine and shape and bake it as directed in the recipe.

10. Remove the ring from the oven, sift the powdered sugar over the top, and serve warm.

NUTRITIONAL FACTS (PER SERVING)

Calories: 138   Carbohydrate: 29 g   Cholesterol: 0 mg
Fat: 1.9 g   Fiber: 1.7 g   Protein: 4 g   Sodium: 59 mg

DIABETIC EXCHANGES: 1 Starch, 1 Fruit

Cherry-Cheese Loaf

Yield: 14 slices

1 recipe Whole Wheat Sweet Dough (page 151)

2 teaspoons skim milk

2 tablespoons sliced toasted almonds (page 87)

FILLING

1 block (8 ounces) nonfat cream cheese

1 egg white, or 2 tablespoons fat-free egg substitute

2 tablespoons unbleached flour

1 teaspoon vanilla extract

Sugar substitute equal to $\frac{1}{4}$ cup sugar (page 19)

1 cup canned light (reduced-sugar) cherry pie filling

GLAZE

$\frac{1}{3}$ cup powdered sugar

$1\frac{1}{2}$ teaspoons skim milk

$\frac{1}{4}$ teaspoon vanilla extract

1. To make the filling, place the cream cheese, egg white, flour, vanilla extract, and sugar substitute in a medium-sized bowl. Using an electric mixer, beat the mixture until smooth. Set aside.

2. Place the dough on a lightly floured surface, and, using a rolling pin, roll it into a 10-x-14-inch rectangle. Coat a large baking sheet with nonstick cooking spray, and transfer the dough to the sheet.

3. Using a sharp knife, make $3\frac{1}{4}$-inch-long cuts at 1-inch intervals on both of the 14-inch sides. Spread the cheese filling down the center third of the dough; then cover the cheese mixture with the cherry pie filling. Fold the strips diagonally over the filling, overlapping them to create a braided look. (See the figures on page 148 for clarification.)

4. Cover the loaf with a clean kitchen towel, and let rise in a warm place for about 45 minutes, or until doubled in size.

5. Lightly brush the top of the loaf with the skim milk. Bake at 350°F for about 22 minutes, or until the loaf is lightly browned. Remove from the oven and let sit for about 3 minutes.

6. To make the glaze, combine all of the glaze ingredients in a small bowl, and stir until smooth. Drizzle the glaze over the warm loaf, and sprinkle with the almonds. Serve warm.

NUTRITIONAL FACTS (PER SLICE)

Calories: 126   Carbohydrate: 24.5 g   Cholesterol: 1 mg
Fat: 0.4 g   Fiber: 1.3 g   Protein: 5.5 g   Sodium: 169 mg

DIABETIC EXCHANGES: 1 Starch, $\frac{2}{3}$ Fruit

Apricot-Pecan Bread

Yield: 24 slices

1 cup chopped dried apricots

1 cup boiling water

2 cups whole wheat pastry flour

1 teaspoon baking powder

1 teaspoon baking soda

¼ cup plus 2 tablespoons honey

¼ cup evaporated skimmed milk

2 teaspoons vanilla extract

⅔ cup chopped pecans

1. Place the apricots in a medium-sized bowl, and pour the boiling water over the fruit. Set the mixture aside until it has cooled to room temperature.

2. Place the flour, baking powder, and baking soda in a large bowl, and stir to mix well. Add the apricot mixture, including the water, and the honey, milk, and vanilla extract, and stir just until the dry ingredients are moistened. Fold in the pecans.

3. Coat three 1-pound cans with nonstick cooking spray. Divide the batter evenly among the cans, and bake at 300°F for about 40 minutes, or just until a wooden toothpick inserted in the center of a loaf comes out clean.

4. Remove the bread from the oven, and let sit for 10 minutes. Invert the loaves onto a wire rack, turn right side up, and cool to room temperature. Wrap the loaves in aluminum foil or plastic wrap, and let sit overnight before slicing and serving. (Overnight storage will give the loaves a softer, moister crust.)

NUTRITIONAL FACTS (PER SLICE)

Calories: 86   Carbohydrate: 15 g   Cholesterol: 0 mg
Fat: 2.3 g   Fiber: 1.8 g   Protein: 2 g   Sodium: 70 mg

DIABETIC EXCHANGES: ½ Starch, ½ Fruit, ½ Fat

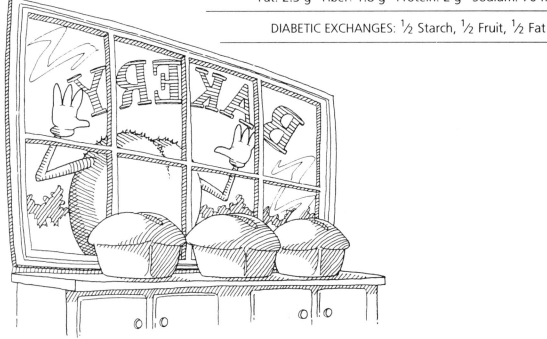

Apple Streusel Bread

1. To make the filling, place the apples, $\frac{1}{2}$ cup of the juice, and the cinnamon and raisins or cranberries in a $1\frac{1}{2}$-quart pot, and bring to a boil over high heat. Reduce the heat to medium-low and cover. Stirring occasionally, simmer for 5 minutes, or until the apples are soft.

2. Place the remaining 2 tablespoons of apple juice and the cornstarch in a small bowl, and stir to dissolve the cornstarch. Add the cornstarch mixture to the apple mixture, and cook, stirring constantly, for about 1 minute, or until thick and bubbly. Remove the pot from the heat, and allow to cool to room temperature. Stir in the sugar substitute.

3. Place the dough on a lightly floured surface, and, using a rolling pin, roll it into a 10-x-14-inch rectangle. Coat a large baking sheet with nonstick cooking spray, and transfer the dough to the sheet.

4. Using a sharp knife, make $3\frac{1}{4}$-inch-long cuts at 1-inch intervals on both of the 14-inch sides. Spread the cooled filling down the center third of the dough. Fold the strips diagonally over the filling, overlapping the strips to create a braided look. (See the figures on page 148 for clarification.)

5. Cover the loaf with a clean kitchen towel, and let rise in a warm place for about 45 minutes, or until doubled in size.

6. Lightly brush the top of the loaf with the skim milk. To make the streusel topping, combine the flour and brown sugar in a small bowl. Using a pastry cutter or 2 knives, cut the margarine or butter into the flour mixture until crumbly. Stir in the nuts, and sprinkle the topping over the loaf.

7. Bake at 350°F for about 22 minutes, or until the loaf is lightly browned. Serve warm.

Yield: 14 slices

1 recipe Whole Wheat Sweet Dough (page 151)

2 teaspoons skim milk

FILLING

3 cups chopped peeled apples

$\frac{1}{2}$ cup plus 2 tablespoons apple juice, divided

$\frac{1}{2}$ teaspoon ground cinnamon

$\frac{1}{2}$ cup dark raisins or dried cranberries

1 tablespoon plus 1 teaspoon cornstarch

Sugar substitute equal to 2 tablespoons sugar (page 19)

TOPPING

2 tablespoons whole wheat pastry flour

2 tablespoons light brown sugar

1 tablespoon reduced-fat margarine or light butter, cut into pieces

3 tablespoons finely chopped walnuts

NUTRITIONAL FACTS (PER SLICE)

Calories: 158   Carbohydrate: 33 g   Cholesterol: 0 mg
Fat: 1.9 g   Fiber: 2.2 g   Protein: 3.6 g   Sodium: 93 mg

DIABETIC EXCHANGES: 1 Starch, 1 Fruit

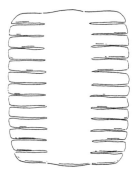

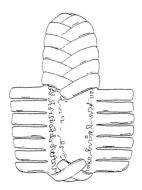

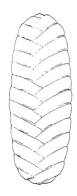

a. Make 3¼-inch-long cuts at 1-inch intervals on each side of the dough.

b. Fold the dough strips diagonally over the filling.

c. Continue folding the strips to create a "braided" loaf.

Making Apple Streusel Bread.

Cinnamon-Raisin Ring

Yield: 16 slices

1 recipe Whole Wheat Sweet Dough (page 151)

2 teaspoons skim milk

FILLING

3 tablespoons maple syrup

½ teaspoon ground cinnamon

½ cup dark raisins

⅓ cup chopped walnuts

GLAZE

⅓ cup powdered sugar

1¾ teaspoons skim milk

⅛ teaspoon ground cinnamon

1. Place the dough on a lightly floured surface, and, using a rolling pin, roll it into a 11-x-16-inch rectangle. Combine the maple syrup and cinnamon in a small dish, and spread the mixture over the dough to within ½ inch of the edges. Sprinkle the raisins and nuts over the syrup. Roll the rectangle up jelly roll-style, beginning at the long end.

2. Coat a baking sheet with nonstick spray, and place the roll on the pan, bringing the ends around to form a circle. Using scissors, cut almost all of the way through the dough at 1-inch intervals. Twist each 1-inch segment to turn the cut side up. Cover with a kitchen towel, and let rise in a warm place for 25 minutes, or until doubled in size.

3. Lightly brush the top of the ring with the 2 teaspoons of skim milk. Bake at 350°F for about 15 minutes, or until lightly browned. Remove from the oven and allow to cool for about 3 minutes.

4. To make the glaze, combine the glaze ingredients in a small bowl, stirring until smooth. Drizzle the glaze over the warm ring, and serve.

NUTRITIONAL FACTS (PER SLICE)
Calories: 134   Carbohydrate: 27 g   Cholesterol: 0 mg
Fat: 1.8 g   Fiber: 1.5 g   Protein: 3.3 g   Sodium: 78 mg

DIABETIC EXCHANGES: 1 Starch, ¾ Fruit, ⅓ Fat

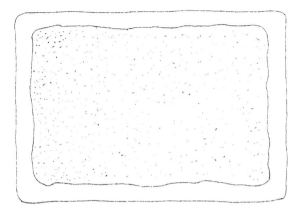

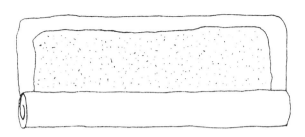

a. Spread the filling over the dough.

b. Roll the dough up jelly-roll style.

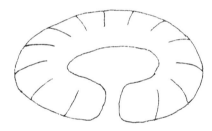

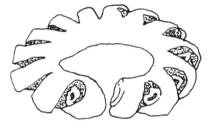

c. Bend the roll into a ring, and cut almost all the way through at 1-inch intervals.

d. Twist each 1-inch segment to turn the cut side up.

Making Cinnamon-Raisin Ring.

Cherry-Almond Ring

Yield: 16 slices

For variety, substitute raspberries or blueberries for the cherries.

1 recipe Whole Wheat Sweet
   Dough (page 151)

2 teaspoons skim milk

2 tablespoons sliced toasted
   almonds (page 87)

FILLING

1 cup chopped pitted frozen
   (unthawed) cherries

3 tablespoons white grape juice,
   divided

1 tablespoon cornstarch

Sugar substitute equal to $\frac{1}{4}$ cup
   sugar (page 19)

GLAZE

$\frac{1}{3}$ cup powdered sugar

1$\frac{1}{2}$ teaspoons skim milk

$\frac{1}{4}$ teaspoon almond extract

1. To prepare the filling, place the cherries and 2 tablespoons of the juice in a small saucepan, and bring to a boil over medium-high heat. Reduce the heat to low, cover, and cook for about 4 minutes, or until the cherries are soft.

2. Place the remaining tablespoon of juice and the cornstarch in a small dish, and stir to dissolve the cornstarch. Add the cornstarch mixture to the cherries, and cook and stir for another minute or 2, or until thick and bubbly. Remove the pot from the heat, and allow to cool to room temperature. Stir in the sugar substitute.

3. Place the dough on a lightly floured surface, and, using a rolling pin, roll it into an 11-x-16-inch rectangle. Spread the filling over the dough to within $\frac{1}{2}$ inch of the edges, and roll the rectangle up jelly roll-style, beginning at the long end.

4. Coat a large baking sheet with nonstick cooking spray, and place the roll on the pan, bringing the ends around to form a circle. Using scissors, cut almost all of the way through the dough at 1-inch intervals. Twist each 1-inch segment to turn the cut side up. (See the figures on page 149 for clarification.) Cover with a clean kitchen towel, and let rise in a warm place for about 35 minutes, or until doubled in size.

5. Lightly brush the top of the ring with the 2 teaspoons of skim milk. Bake at 350°F for about 15 minutes, or until lightly browned. Remove from the oven and let sit for about 3 minutes.

6. To make the glaze, combine all of the glaze ingredients in a small bowl, and stir until smooth. Drizzle the glaze over the warm ring, and sprinkle with the almonds. Serve immediately.

NUTRITIONAL FACTS (PER SLICE)

Calories: 107   Carbohydrate: 22.5 g   Cholesterol: 0 mg
Fat: 0.7 g   Fiber: 1.3 g   Protein: 2.7 g   Sodium: 78 mg

DIABETIC EXCHANGES: 1 Starch, $\frac{1}{2}$ Fruit

A Dough for All Seasons

Warm, fragrant, and delicious, sweet yeast breads, coffee cakes, and buns are always a special treat. And with just one sweet dough recipe, you can make an infinite number of tantalizing baked goods. Use Whole Wheat Sweet Dough to prepare some of the yeast dessert breads presented in this chapter, or draw upon your imagination to create your own cinnamon rolls, coffee cakes, buns, and breads.

If the thought of making yeast dough from scratch scares you, fear not. This recipe is easily mixed by hand. Or, if you own a bread machine, follow the simple instructions provided at the end of the recipe to prepare this versatile dough with a minimum of fuss.

Whole Wheat Sweet Dough

1. Place the water, yeast, and 1 teaspoon of the sugar in a small bowl, and stir to dissolve the yeast. Set aside.

2. Place the remaining sugar, ¾ cup of the unbleached flour, and all of the whole wheat flour and salt in a large bowl, and stir to mix well.

3. Add the yeast mixture and the buttermilk to the flour mixture, and stir for 1 minute. Add 2 tablespoons of the remaining unbleached flour to the dough, and stir to mix. Stir in enough of the remaining flour, 2 tablespoons at a time, to form a stiff dough.

4. Sprinkle 2 tablespoons of the remaining unbleached flour onto a flat surface, and turn the dough onto the surface. Knead the dough for 5 minutes, gradually adding enough of the remaining flour to form a smooth, satiny ball.

5. Coat a large bowl with nonstick cooking spray, and place the dough in the bowl. Cover the bowl with a clean kitchen towel, and let rise in a warm place for about 1 hour, or until doubled in size. Then proceed to shape, fill, and bake the dough according to recipe directions.

Yield: about 1 pound, or 16 servings

¼ cup warm water (105°F–115°F)

2 teaspoons Rapid Rise yeast

¼ cup sugar, divided

2 cups unbleached flour

¾ cup whole wheat pastry flour

½ teaspoon salt

½ cup plus 2 tablespoons nonfat or low-fat buttermilk, warmed to room temperature

NUTRITIONAL FACTS (PER SERVING)

Calories: 85   Carbohydrate: 18 g   Cholesterol: 0 mg
Fat: 0.3 g   Fiber: 1.1 g   Protein: 2.5 g   Sodium: 77 mg

DIABETIC EXCHANGES: 1 Starch

To make Whole Wheat Sweet Dough in a bread machine, simply place all of the dough ingredients except for ¼ cup of the unbleached flour in the machine's bread pan. Turn the machine to the "rise," "dough," "manual," or equivalent setting so the machine will mix, knead, and let the dough rise once.

Check the dough about 5 minutes after the machine has started. If the dough seems too sticky, add more of the remaining flour, a tablespoon at a time. When the dough is ready, remove it from the machine and proceed to shape, fill, and bake it as directed in the recipe of your choice.

Cranberry-Orange Ring

Yield: 16 servings

1 recipe Whole Wheat Sweet
  Dough (page 151)

2 teaspoons skim milk

1 tablespoon finely chopped
  pecans

FILLING

1 cup fresh or frozen (unthawed)
  cranberries

½ cup chopped dates

¼ cup orange juice

¼ cup chopped pecans

Brown sugar substitute equal to 2
  tablespoons brown sugar
  (page 19)

GLAZE

⅓ cup powdered sugar

1 tablespoon frozen (thawed)
  orange juice concentrate

1. To make the filling, combine the cranberries, dates, and orange juice in a small saucepan, and bring to a boil over high heat. Reduce the heat to medium-low and cover. Stirring occasionally, cook for about 5 minutes, or until the berries have popped and the mixture is thick. Remove the pot from the heat, stir in the pecans and sugar substitute, and allow to cool to room temperature.

2. Place the dough on a lightly floured surface and, using a rolling pin, roll it into a 9-x-18-inch rectangle. Using a knife or pizza wheel, cut the rectangle into 3 strips, each measuring 3 x 18 inches.

3. Lay 1 of the strips on a flat surface so that 1 of the long sides is nearest you. Spread a third of the filling in a line along the bottom of the strip. Moisten the top edge of the strip lightly with water. Then roll up the strip from the bottom, enclosing the filling. Pinch the dough along the seam to seal. Repeat this procedure with the remaining strips and filling.

4. Place the rolled strips alongside one another, with the seam sides down. Braid the strips together. Bring the ends of the strips together to form a ring, and pinch the ends together to seal.

5. Coat a 9-inch round cake pan with nonstick cooking spray, and place the ring in the pan. Cover with a clean kitchen towel, and let rise in a warm place for about 1 hour, or until doubled in size.

6. Brush the top of the ring with the skim milk, and bake at 350°F for about 22 minutes, or until lightly browned. Remove from the oven and allow to cool for about 3 minutes.

7. To make the glaze, combine the glaze ingredients in a small bowl, and stir until smooth. Drizzle the glaze over the warm ring, and sprinkle with the pecans. Serve warm.

NUTRITIONAL FACTS (PER SLICE)
Calories: 130   Carbohydrate: 26 g   Cholesterol: 0 mg
Fat: 1.9 g   Fiber: 1.9 g   Protein: 2.8 g   Sodium: 78 mg

DIABETIC EXCHANGES: 1 Starch, ¾ Fruit

Resource List

Most of the ingredients used in the recipes in this book are readily available in any supermarket, or can be found in your local health foods store or gourmet shop. But if you are unable to locate what you're looking for, the following list should guide you to a manufacturer who can either sell the desired product to you directly or inform you of the nearest retail outlet.

Whole Grains and Flours

Arrowhead Mills, Inc.
Box 2059
Hereford, TX 79045
(800) 749-0730

Whole wheat pastry flour, oat flour, and other flours and whole grains.

King Arthur Flour
PO Box 876
Norwich, VT 05055
(800) 827-6836

White whole wheat flour, whole wheat pastry flour, unbleached pastry flour, and other flours, whole grains, and baking products.

Mountain Ark Trading Company
PO Box 3170
Fayetteville, AR 72702
(800) 643-8909

Whole grains and flours, unrefined sweeteners, dried fruits, fruit spreads, and a wide variety of other natural foods.

Walnut Acres
PO Box 8
Penns Creek, PA 17862
(800) 433-3998

Baking and cooking aids, whole grains, whole grain flours, unrefined sweeteners, dried fruits, and a wide variety of other natural foods.

Sweeteners

Advanced Ingredients
331 Capitola Avenue, Suite F
Capitola, CA 95010
(408) 464-9891

Fruit Source granulated and liquid sweeteners.

Sucanat North America Corporation
26 Clinton Drive #117
Hollis, NH 03049
(603) 595-2922

Sucanat granulated sweetener.

Vermont Country Maple, Inc.
76 Ethan Allen Drive
South Burlington, VT 05403
(800) 528-7021

Maple sugar, maple syrup, and other maple products.

Index